BECOMING A
CONSUMMATE CLINICIAN

Hospital Medicine: Current Concepts

Scott A. Flanders and Sanjay Saint, *Series Editors*

BECOMING A CONSUMMATE CLINICIAN

What Every Student, House Officer, and Hospital Practitioner Needs to Know

Ary L. Goldberger, M.D.

Professor of Medicine
Harvard Medical School and
Wyss Institute for Biologically Inspired Engineering at Harvard University
Director, Margret and H.A. Rey Institute for Nonlinear Dynamics in Medicine
Beth Israel Deaconess Medical Center
Boston, MA

Zachary D. Goldberger, M.D., M.S.

Assistant Professor of Medicine
Division of Cardiology
Harborview Medical Center
University of Washington School of Medicine
Seattle, WA

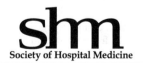

Society of Hospital Medicine

Hospitalists. Transforming Healthcare.
Revolutionizing Patient Care.

⊛WILEY-BLACKWELL

A JOHN WILEY & SONS, INC., PUBLICATION

Published by John Wiley & Sons, Inc., Hoboken, New Jersey
Published simultaneously in Canada

For general information on our other products and services or for technical support, please contact our Customer Care Department within the United States at (800) 762-2974, outside the United States at (317) 572-3993 or fax (317) 572-4002.

Wiley also publishes its books in a variety of electronic formats. Some content that appears in print may not be available in electronic formats. For more information about Wiley products, visit our web site at www.wiley.com.

Library of Congress Cataloging-in-Publication Data:

Goldberger, Ary Louis, 1949–
   Becoming a consummate clinician : what every student, house officer, and hospital practitioner needs to know / Ary L. Goldberger, Zachary D. Goldberger.
      p. ; cm. – (Hospital medicine: current concept ; 3)
      ISBN 978-1-118-01143-0 (pbk.)
   I. Goldberger, Zachary D.   II. Title.   III. Series: Hospital medicine, current concepts ; 3.
   [DNLM: 1. Clinical Medicine.   2. Evidence-Based Medicine.   3. Interprofessional Relations.   4. Medical Errors–prevention & control.   5. Teaching Rounds–methods. WB 102]
      610.73–dc23

                                                                                    2012023634

Printed in the United States of America

10 9 8 7 6 5 4 3 2 1

For
Erin, Ellen, and Nicki
Annabel, Tabitha, and Quinn
and for Lexy

CONTENTS

PART 2   MEDICAL MASTERIES

PREFACE

You've had the usual busy day. Just finished seeing and writing up the last of six patients admitted overnight to your service (including one who had to be transferred to the ICU with sepsis). Sent in an application to the medical center's curriculum committee for a proposed new course, "The Golden Glove: Defining, Detecting, and Eradicating Medical Errors." Late for a hospital committee meeting on the new quality initiative to improve care in postoperative patients.

When you return to your office, two of the 59 new e-mails in your inbox catch your eye. The first is from a third-year medical student who presents with the complaint that "I feel disoriented and confused only one day after starting my medical clerkship." This note is not a request for a neurological consult but, rather, a distress signal from one of your mentees who has been touching base with you throughout her clinical years without any indication of prior problems.

The second e-mail, from a friend and colleague, says: "Work and teaching rounds took four hours today! How can we teach students and house officers to present more clearly and concisely and how to frame a differential diagnosis?"

This book is written for hyper-busy clinicians/teachers and their trainees who face these types of challenges related to apparent gaps between the world of the class and the world of the wards. Despite the best-intended efforts of courses with names such as "The Doctor–Patient Encounter," students and their preceptors often express the sense that essential but hard-to-identify components are missing from our training efforts. These missing links contribute to the types of frustrations voiced above. We have adopted the term *interstitial curriculum* as a way of defining selected necessary concepts and practices that seem to fall between the disciplinary cracks of contemporary medical education programs.

Throughout the book, we highlight these concepts with mini-case examples. Most are drawn from internal medicine; further, a cardiovascular bias will unmask the specialty orientation of the authors, but hopefully will not prove limiting.

The complementary processes of constantly rethinking assumptions, researching information, and reformulating basic mechanisms are fundamental to practicing all types of medicine successfully. Such processes also help to avoid potentially lethal errors and help to rigorously and compassionately advance the inseparable sciences of prevention and healing. These deep and multidimensional challenges are central to the ongoing pursuit of becoming the consummate clinician.

ARY L. GOLDBERGER
ZACHARY D. GOLDBERGER

ACKNOWLEDGMENTS

We wish to acknowledge our many students, colleagues, and patients over the years, and the many others who inspired this short book. Finding oneself adrift in a turbulent clinical sea midway through medical school is, to say the least, daunting. Finding others with similar questions and existential anxieties is therapeutic, but what we really want are the keys to the kingdom where medical house staff and residents seem to speak that mysterious dialect of *clinicalese* with high fluency, and possess apparently uncanny reasoning and communication skills. Having read the same textbooks, taken similar preclinical lectures, and passed similar exams, we wondered whether we had all inadvertently missed some extracurricular but essential mentoring sessions somewhere along the way. Could this bridging knowledge be restored?

The discovery that the classroom-to-clinic gap was more the rule than the exception became a prime motivator for writing the book. Many people played important roles, including students at Yale School of Medicine, University of California–San Diego, University of Washington, Harvard Medical School, and University of Michigan.

A number of colleagues have read sections and have offered important critical reviews. Among those are our wives, Erin Fouch, M.D., and Ellen Goldberger, J.D., and colleagues, Tom Delbanco, M.D., Richard Schwartzstein, M.D., Vikas Sukhatme, M.D., Ph.D.,

Michael Volk, M.D., M.S., Colin R. Cooke, M.D., M.Sc., and Madalena Costa, Ph.D.

Zachary D. Goldberger would like to offer special thanks to Drs. Rod Hayward, Caroline Richardson, and Sandeep Vijan for their methodological instruction and to Drs. Michael Shea, Daniel Eitzman, and David Coleman for their superb clinical mentorship.

Zachary D. Goldberger was supported by a grant from the Robert Wood Johnson Foundation Clinical Scholars Program while writing this book and Ary L. Goldberger by a grant from the G. Harold and Leila Y. Mathers Charitable Foundation. However, the views expressed do not necessarily reflect those of either foundation.

Our intrepid editor at Wiley-Blackwell, Thom Moore, and his assistant Ian Collins, played key roles in shaping the material and in inviting us to join the Hospital Medicine book series edited by Scott Flanders and Sanjay Saint.

However, we take full responsibility for any errors, and the gratitude expressed to our critical readers in no way indicates their agreement or endorsement. If the lessons of this text are crafted successfully, readers will critically rethink what we say here as well as everything else they read. We also recognize that some of the topics and their presentations are not without general controversy and urge our readers to contact us via the publisher or through e-mail if they wish. Even better, discuss these issues on rounds.

Finally, we note that the process of becoming a consummate clinician is never-ending and rarely predictable. This book is a guide to clinically perplexed trainees and their attendings. On your unique and unforgettable journeys, we wish you grand luck—the serendipity that favors the well-prepared, but not overly rehearsed mind.

ALG
ZDG

SURVIVING AND THRIVING IN WARD WORLD

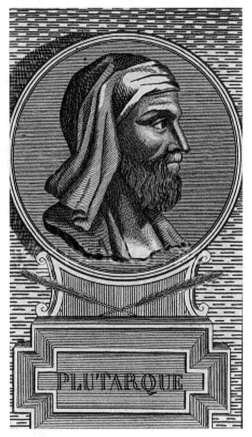

Plutarch, a first-century Greek moralist.

Becoming a Consummate Clinician: What Every Student, House Officer, and Hospital Practitioner Needs to Know, First Edition.
Ary L. Goldberger and Zachary D. Goldberger.
© 2012 Wiley-Blackwell. Published 2012 by John Wiley & Sons, Inc.

The mind is not a vessel to be filled but a fire to be kindled.
                                          —PLUTARCH (ca. A.D. 46–120)

The most important failure was one of imagination.
        —THE 9/11 COMMISSION REPORT: The National Commission on
    Terrorist Attacks on the United States; General Findings, Section 509

This book addresses a number of audiences. For clinical clerks and
house officers, it is intended as a springboard or launching pad to
help them hit the ground running on the wards. We hope to provide
some immediately applicable tips and to guide trainees in avoiding
common pitfalls and pratfalls of gathering, processing, and communicating medical information. For more experienced hospital-based
practitioners, hopefully it will provide an organizing framework for
coping with some of the daily challenges in both patient care and
mentoring that somehow escape mention in lengthier texts.

> For trainees, who readily and understandably feel lost in their early rotations,
> this is also intended as a kind of clinical GPS—a way of helping you locate
> and track your clinical coordinates and keep your bearings in the face of
> major new challenges and the inherent uncertainties of clinical medicine.

What/how should I be thinking upon hearing the following chief
complaints? What does an experienced, active clinical listener actually think?

- A 30-year-old man presents with a fainting spell.
- A 60-year-old woman presents with shortness of breath.

Part 1 (Chapters 1 to 6) is called *Medical Musts and Must-Nots*.
These discussions are geared toward more basic and essential issues
(the must-knows) of information gathering from the history and
physical exam, as well as formulating differential diagnoses. Special
emphasis is given to avoiding common mistakes and offering tips
toward achieving the clinical savvy of more experienced physicians.
These chapters also include perspectives from the attending's side:

how to listen to and interact with presentations by team members and enhance the teaching value of rounds.

Part 2 (Chapters 7 to 12) is called *Medical Masteries*. Leveraging off the material in Part 1, these chapters deal with aspects of critical analysis of medical data and invite a reexamination of some of the ways we "think about thinking" in clinical medicine. Topics include reducing medical errors, revisiting evidence-based medicine, deconstructing Sutton's "law" and other widely cited medical aphorisms, the perils of a major but rarely discussed source of medical bias (semantic bias), and transforming information and knowledge into deeper understanding.

In Chapter 12 we examine two central and coupled questions for students and attendings that are almost never asked in the formal medical school curriculum: "What is health?" and "What is disease?" These omissions are remarkable given that two central goals of medicine are devoted to maintaining and restoring the former, and to curing or palliating the latter, both in practice and in research.

Another provocative question that helped to motivate this book was posed by a non-M.D. colleague: Is there a way for medical students and others to "get inside the heads" of their more experienced clinical mentors, short of being an actual apprentice? As in every other aspect of our professional lives, no substitute exists for real-world clinical experience and expert tutelage. But realistic recognition of the limitations of any enterprise is not a statement of its futility.

The good news for students is that certain general principles of clinical thinking and practice–what we call the *interstitial curriculum*– although not the substance of most textbook presentations, can be taught as part of a type of a *facilitated apprenticeship* toward clinical mastery. Further, some of these essentials can be conveyed concisely in guidebook form, especially to those who already have some medical background or interest.

We emphasize that the term *interstitial curriculum*—what's not explicitly taught but should be—is *not* to be confused with the *hidden curriculum*, a subject that is receiving increasing attention. The latter refers to the unspoken biases that warp both medical and nonmedical education (i.e., what shouldn't be taught but somehow is). For doctors, the hidden curriculum has been used, for example, to describe the disparaging and nonempathic behavior that students and trainees may absorb from their seniors. Readers interested in the applications of the hidden curriculum in medical education are referred to the literature, with selected references given in the bibliography.

THREE KEY CHALLENGES FOR STUDENTS AND PRACTITIONERS

Three central and closely related challenges for every practitioner of medicine at all levels, from student to senior hospitalist attending, are:

1. *To enrich the way we think* about diagnosis, therapy, and prognosis, especially at the warp speed of ward world, which increasingly lurches between the frazzled and the frantic.
2. *To enhance our communication skills*: developing good habits for presenting information and preventing or curing some counterproductive habits.
3. *To help reduce, and to the extent possible, eradicate medical errors.* Asking some relatively simple questions as a routine part of self-examination during rounds can literally transform an entire hospital's systems for the better.

Learning and practicing critical thinking skills that often resist conventional wisdom, actively looking for anomalous findings (making "outlier" rounds), and harnessing the energies of imagination are essential components of clinical medicine and powerful antidotes to cognitive errors (Chapter 7). From a more positive perspective, the combination of critical plus imaginative thinking is the source of successful therapeutic interventions and clinical discoveries. Helping students and trainees acquire and master these skills and render them in a compassionate manner are perhaps the most challenging goals in medical didactics. For busy practitioner-mentors, in particular, not losing touch with foundational attributes and being able to transmit these skills is one of the most demanding aspects of medical education, and one most at risk in the age of information overload and "high-throughput" patient care.

UNCOMPLICATING LIFE IN A COMPLEX WORLD

The nature of critical thinking essential to bedside and basic medicine is also much more general and applies to coping with virtually all *complex systems* where prediction, diagnosis, forecasting, and prevention are always at play. The words "at play" may seem ill-chosen for such a daunting and serious set of obligations. Yet the stunning "failure of imagination" critique in the 9/11 Commission Report indicates a dearth of creativity—a lack of general inventiveness that informs the best science and promotes optimal ways of protecting society at large and its members. An unexpected link between the terrorist attacks of 9/11 and one aspect of public health— risk of sudden death in areas outside the lower Manhattan explosion sites—is described briefly in Chapter 12.

THE

9/11

COMMISSION

REPORT

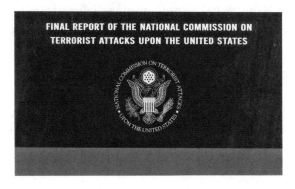

FINAL REPORT OF THE NATIONAL COMMISSION ON
TERRORIST ATTACKS UPON THE UNITED STATES

Although we cannot predict future events and discoveries, we can anticipate that the rate of information expansion will continue at a lightning (if not always enlightening) pace. Indeed, Moore's law, proposed in 1975, famously posited that the number of transistors placed on integrated circuits will double about every two years for the foreseeable future. This exponential growth of microprocessing capacity, resulting in smaller and smaller and less expensive computers, is related to the expanding amounts and accessibility of information, including biomedical data. Whether Moore's prediction turns out be a law or more of a useful approximation, it is certainly more relevant to medicine than Sutton's Law (Chapter 10). But our point here is that the continuing explosion of computer processing capability and with it of information/data, captured in Moore's provocative prediction, does not neatly translate into knowledge or understanding on the wards. Indeed, as noted above, information/data overload can, paradoxically, imperil creative and critical thinking.

We can only anticipate one thing with great certainty: that the future will always include surprises—*expect the unexpected*. This "certainty of uncertainty" law compels the need for flexible cognitive infrastructures and strategies for handling and making the most of the information available. Exercising and refining cognitive tools are essential to clinical success, just as adaptability and plasticity are fundamental to the health of ecosystems, species, and individuals. Indeed, the best intended efforts to codify clinical judgment into clinical rules (even if only intended as guidelines) and the development of ever more sophisticated algorithmic trees are inherently limited. Furthermore, such efforts sometimes undermine efforts to foster the desired three R's of rigor, rationality, and reliability central to evidence-based medical practice.

UNEXPECTED INNOVATION

The fortuitous discovery of penicillin, the first antibiotic, by the Scottish bacteriologist Alexander Fleming on September 3, 1928, is one of the best examples of Louis Pasteur's dictum: "Chance favors the prepared mind." Fleming had just returned to his laboratory in London after a vacation. He had been culturing *Staphylococcus aureus* and was discarding petri dishes from leftover experiments. He looked down and noticed that one of his cultures was contaminated with mold. A clear area around the mold caught his eye and prompted him to surmise that the contaminant was secreting a bactericidal substance. With the help of a colleague, Fleming grew a pure culture of what is now known to be *Penicillium notatum*.

This account has been embellished and even mythologized to a certain extent, but these facts seem reasonably solid. Also of note is that the purification and characterization of the compound and, shortly thereafter, the mass production of penicillin—what we would call the *translational medicine* aspects—did not occur until years later. Like many discoveries, Fleming's breakthrough was not part of a carefully crafted game plan, any more than the discovery of x-rays or magnetic resonance followed a linear path from original design to bedside applications. Quite the opposite—these triumphs of translational medicine were not motivated by or even initially connected to the practice of medicine. Instead, scientific, including clinical, creativity most often erupts unexpectedly from a combination of intuition, imagination, and observation, combined with intellectual rigor and a special type of fearless intensity. Sir Isaac Newton commented: "An essential aspect of creativity is not being afraid to fail."

For students and trainees of medicine, as well as their mentors, the wards offer perhaps the richest—and sometimes the most intimidating—precincts for discovery and learning, which can transform the lives of single patients and entire groups. But to make these contributions (e.g, preventing a potentially lethal drug–drug interaction in a patient on your first rotation on the wards and then helping to set up fail-safe measures for others) requires that you first overcome the daunting gap between the preclinical and clinical worlds.

Mini-summary and Preview: Perhaps the most difficult challenges faced by practitioners of medicine at all levels are those that deal with navigating the gap between the classroom and the clinic, between the textbook pages we read and the urgent text pages we receive.

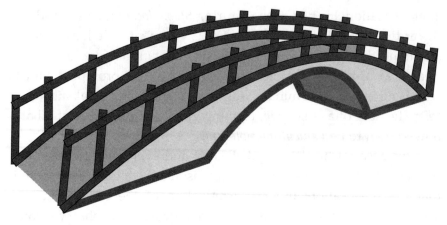

Bridge the classroom-to-clinic gap.

After the first day of their medical clerkships, students may be left wondering:

- What happened to the textbook tables and electronic guides that describe how clinicians think about diagnoses?
- Why didn't someone tell me how cases are really presented on rounds? (Their hospital-based attendings and house officers also ask the same question.)
- Why don't the algorithms for the diagnosis and treatment of a given condition account for the individual patient I am treating?
- Why did the drug listed under "antiarrhythmics to treat atrial fibrillation" in our pharmacology book induce a cardiac arrest in my patient? How can elegantly targeted therapy to treat diabetes or certain forms of cancer land so far off-target?
- What actually is evidence-based medicine, and where is the evidence?

The goal of the 12 chapters ahead is to invite students, house officers, and their more senior colleagues to rethink basic issues that previously may have seemed self-evident and even trivial (e.g., gravity before Newton, or the inevitability of infections before modern medicine). These challenges turn out to be deep and multi-dimensional. Most important to busy students and practitioners is that these challenges have enormous practical ramifications for critical thinking, basic research, and bedside patient care.

MEDICAL MUSTS AND MUST-NOTS: SIX ESSENTIALS OF WARD WORLD

CHAPTER 1

HOW (NOT) TO PRESENT A PATIENT HISTORY

Only connect. . . .

—E.M. Forster (1879–1970), *Howards End*

A doctor who cannot take a good history and a patient who cannot give one are in danger of giving and receiving bad treatment.
—Anonymous, quoted by Paul Dudley White, M.D.,
in *Clues in the Diagnosis and Treatment of Heart Disease* (1956)

For students, either you have already discovered, or will soon learn, that delivering a medical presentation on rounds is a challenging and sometimes terrifying experience. You have to satisfy two conflicting sets of goals simultaneously: accuracy and comprehensiveness vs. succinctness and efficiency.

THE HIDDEN HISTORY OF A HISTORY

It is surprising how ineffectively and inefficiently many physicians, especially those in training, communicate clinical information. Clinical savvy, technical skills, and communication skills are not

Becoming a Consummate Clinician: What Every Student, House Officer, and Hospital Practitioner Needs to Know, First Edition.
Ary L. Goldberger and Zachary D. Goldberger.
© 2012 Wiley-Blackwell. Published 2012 by John Wiley & Sons, Inc.

necessarily positively correlated. A reliable sign of this problem is the *restless legs syndrome* or *flamingo sign* (shifting of weight from one leg to the other) observable in colleagues visibly chomping at the bit to move on during seemingly endless presentations.

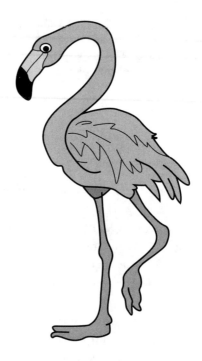

For attendings, presentations by students and house officers can also be anxiety-provoking. As the ultimately responsible physicians, they need to integrate the information they hear, separate signal from noise, and figure out what may have been left out and what may be inaccurate. These pressures are magnified by the time urgencies imposed by high-volume case loads, work hour restrictions, and unavoidable multitasking demands. In addition, rounds are a major component of teaching; employing case material in clinically effective and creative ways is one of the great challenges of clinical didactics.

Clinical Rounds and Case Presentations. Following is the flow of information recommended in initial case presentations:

- Chief complaint
- History (all elements)
- Current medications
- Physical examination
- Data: laboratory/imaging/other diagnostics
- Impressions/assessment: diagnoses/differential diagnoses
- Plans and medical decision making

Clinical rounds can serve at least six major purposes:

1. To review, convey, and share information obtained about patients in a comprehensive, yet concise way.
2. To make diagnostic, therapeutic, and related management decisions and plans based on this information as part of a care-giving team.
3. To identify key information that is not available, and to formulate plans to acquire, if possible, the relevant data that fill in the gaps or resolve inconsistencies.
4. To convey information in an understandable and compassionate way to patients and their families.
5. To utilize this experience in the most expansive way for the teaching of trainees.
6. To identify actual or potential medical errors (near-misses) as the basis for reenergizing current corrective and preventive practices, and where necessary, develop new and imaginative ways to eliminate such errors (Chapter 7).

The purpose of this first chapter is to review common pitfalls and how to avoid them in your presentation of information on rounds. In addition, we discuss briefly the presentation of data from the other perspective: that of the hospital-based attending.

Communication problems are especially prevalent in presentations and write-ups by medical students and incipient house officers. However, even more experienced clinicians are not immune to information-conveying "disorders." Eight of the most common pitfalls you will encounter are summarized below. You and your attending are invited to revise and rework this list.

Common Pitfalls in Presentations

1. Overlooking guideposts in the chief complaint (CC).
2. Giving a nonhistorical history of the present illness (HPI).
3. Getting bogged down with too many negatives, and sometimes positives, in the review of systems (ROS), turning this into an exhaustive and exhausting component of the presentation.
4. Recording an incomplete past medical history (PMH), social history (SH), and family history (FH) with gaps in key information, including medication use, exposures, work and travel data, and job stress.
5. Presenting an exhaustive list of past medical history, some of which may be irrelevant to the current admission (i.e., history of a tonsillectomy 70 years ago in an 80-year-old patient admitted with pneumonia).
6. Presenting a jumbled list of medications rather than a concise summary of current and previous drug therapies.
7. Presenting an unbalanced physical exam: excessive negatives and missing data.
8. Providing a zigzag summary of laboratory tests.

A number of elements are required for a complete medical history (Exhibit 1.1). If any of this information is not available or not applicable, you should indicate this fact. Some books list things in different order (e.g., are vaccinations medications or part of health care maintenance?—obviously, they are both). Should sexual risk assessment be part of the past medical history or listed separately? Where should a sleep health history be included? A major challenge is learning which elements of the history are of importance in a given context. For example, the details of which coronary arteries were bypassed at the time of prior cardiac surgery are critical data to present when a patient is admitted for recurrent exertional angina, but not when he

EXHIBIT 1.1 Ingredients of an Adult's Admission History (Narrative)

1. Chief complaint
2. History of present illness
3. Review of systems
4. Past medical history: childhood; surgical evaluations and procedures/operations; adult medical (including hospitalizations); reproductive (for females: menses; pregnancy/obstetric; psychiatric)
5. Medication profile
   (a) Current and prior medications (including herbal/nutritional supplements)
   (b) Allergies (immunologic reactions)
   (c) Nonallergic adverse drug reactions/intolerances (e.g., nausea with erythromycin)
   (d) Recreational or illicit drug use: past and present
6. Personal: habits and health care maintenance
   (a) Dietary and exercise history: include food allergies, restrictions, and special needs
   (b) Tobacco use: past and present (cigarettes, cigars, chewing tobacco, etc.)
   (c) Alcohol: past and present
   (d) Screening procedures (e.g., colonoscopy, etc.)
   (e) Vaccinations
   (f) Injury prevention (e.g., seat belt use)
   (g) Screening for abuse, neglect, or domestic violence
   (h) Sexual risk assessment (including preferences, birth control, sexually transmitted diseases)
   (i) Sleep-related problems (insomnia, loud snoring, daytime somnolence, etc.)
7. Occupational/environmental hazards or exposures (e.g., asbestos, sunburns)
8. Geriatric (as indicated): routine activities of daily living (ADLs): dressing, eating, continence, transfer, toileting, bathing, locomotion, etc.: Instrumental ADLs: shopping, housework, finances, meds, laundry, cooking, etc.
9. Social history: including major relationships and social supports; living arrangements; work status; relevant spiritual and cultural beliefs
10. Family history (including cause and age of death; psychiatric problems)
11. Concerns: financial and insurance-related; impact of illness on job and home life; sexual function; relationships; etc.
12. Advance directive and health care proxy status

is admitted for cellulitis. In the latter case, the oral presentation would still need to note his important history of coronary disease, the status following his uncomplicated bypass surgery four years ago, and the most recent follow-up with his cardiologist.

Next, we discuss four selected aspects of major trouble spots in write-ups and case presentations: the CC, HPI, ROS, and PMH.

Chief Complaints About the Chief Complaint

The chief complaint (CC) sets the tone for the rest of the presentation, analogous to a brief overture to an opera or musical. A major problem with the statement of the CC is a lack of guideposts or pointers. In addition to stating a patient's actual complaint in his or her words— *essential information*—it is helpful to include a few orienting phrases, or *indicators*, to give context to the patient's admission. These phrases do not bias the analysis but, rather, help the listener process extremely complex information.

As with all elements of the presentation, what you actually decide to present on rounds will differ from what is written in your admission note (which should be as complete as possible, as the reader can choose which areas to focus on, but not be burdened with unnecessary detail). Below are two renditions of the CC on three patients that would be found in an admission note or presented orally. The use of a few guidepost qualifiers (shown in italics) is intended to provide useful context to the admission, without creating listener bias.

Case 1: Mr. Kent

> *Version 1:* This is the first Metropolis General Hospital admission for Mr. Clarke Kent, a 60-year-old man with chief complaints of "weakness and fatigue."
>
> *Version 2:* This is the first Metropolis General Hospital admission for Mr. Clarke Kent, a 60-year-old man with *multiple medical and surgical problems* complaining of *increasing* "weakness and fatigue" *for the past month.*

Case 2: Ms. Lane

> *Version 1:* This is the first Metropolis General Hospital admission for Ms. Louise Lane, a 35-year-old woman with a chief complaint of "pain in my belly."
>
> *Version 2:* This is the first Metropolis General Hospital admission for Ms. Louise Lane, a 35-year-old woman with *type 2 diabetes*

with a chief complaint of *intermittent* "belly pain" *starting two days ago.*

Case 3: Mr. Olsen

Version 1: Mr. James Olsen is a 27-year-old man transferred for evaluation of mental status changes.

Version 2: This is the first Metropolis General Hospital admission for Mr. James Olsen, a 27-year-old man transferred *from Apple Community Hospital for further assessment and treatment* of mental status changes. *Mr. Olsen is lethargic and unable to give any specific complaints. Historical details are obtained from his records and his family (sister and brother-in-law), who accompanied him.*

The second versions of the CC are preferable in the three cases since they accomplish three goals: the goals are (1) to be concise, (2) to convey specific information, and (3) to conserve a patient's own words. Using the patient's own words in the CC [patients rarely, if ever, complain of an "FUO" (a fever of unknown origin) or of "atypical chest pain"] is important. For example, a patient who reports "discomfort" or an "ache" or pressure in his chest, representing angina pectoris, may actually deny that he has "chest pain." For physicians, all of these terms may be red flags for symptomatic myocardial ischemia or infarction, but your patient may emphatically resist using the word "pain" even when asked specifically.

History of Present Illness

Two common flaws in presenting a history of the present illness (HPI) are (1) failure to follow a time line—instead, skipping around in a disjointed fashion, and (2) failure to segment the history into subcomplaints when there is a complicated set of problems. As is the case for the CC, you should make a practice of adding *guideposts* and *context* to your recounting of the history. Two patients may both present with abdominal pain; the two statements that follow refer to the same chief complaint but have very different contexts essential to the informed listener:

> *Mrs. Jones's primary complaint of abdominal pain began seven years prior to admission when she was first evaluated and found to have gallstones—cholecystectomy was deferred.*
>
> *Mrs. Jones was feeling fine until one day prior to admission when she developed the acute onset of left lower quadrant pain, which she denies having experienced before.*

The first is about a long chronic history, the second about an apparently acute event.

Not uncommonly, patients will have multiple complaints or their histories will require several concisely summarized subthemes for clarity of presentation. In the example below, the patient has the two concomitant complaints of hyperglycemia and angina pectoris in the context of known diabetes mellitus and coronary disease:

> Diabetes mellitus: *Mr. Stephens has a five-year history of type 2 diabetes formerly treated with diet, and for the last two months with metformin. For the past week, his fasting blood sugars have been persistently higher than what he states is usual.*
>
> Coronary artery disease and chest pain: *Mr. Stephens reports having had no cardiac-type symptoms and a normal treadmill stress test three years prior to admission, performed by his cardiologist, Dr. Lance Palaque. Two years ago the patient developed exertional chest discomfort while shoveling snow. He was admitted to this hospital, and according to our records, had a non-ST elevation myocardial infarction. He underwent cardiac catheterization, which revealed a 90% stenosis in the midportion of the left anterior descending artery, treated with a drug-eluting coronary stent. He now reports one week of exertional chest discomfort similar to his initial symptoms.*

The key indicator of success for history-telling is how well your listeners grasp the essential information in a concise but sufficiently detailed presentation to serve as the basis of management. If you are constantly being interrupted by your attending and team members, you are probably confusing them or leaving out key information. (Or they are just being rude.) The use of notes (e.g., electronic or manual on a 3×5 card) is acceptable, even desirable—but with all records always take care to ensure that HIPAA (Health Insurance and Portability Act) regulations (which serve to protect patient privacy) are being followed (http://www.hhs.gov/ocr/privacy/).

Finally, it is important not to try to convey a specific diagnosis in the history, although one might inadvertently create this type of *formulation bias*. To quote a catch phrase from the classic TV series, *Dragnet*: "Just the facts, ma'am."

A Review of the Review of Systems

The review of systems (ROS) is sometimes mistakenly referred to as the "review of symptoms," which is imprecise since many ingredients of the ROS have nothing to do with symptoms (which are subjective findings). The ROS is equivalent to a comprehensive verbal body scan. A sample inventory of the conventional ROS is given in Exhibit 1.2.

Perhaps the major pitfall in obtaining the ROS is failure to be comprehensive. This shortcoming may be due to lack of time, emergency

EXHIBIT 1.2 Major Ingredients of ROS

General/constitutional
Skin
Breast
Head/eyes/ears/nose/mouth/throat
Cardiovascular
Respiratory
Gastrointestinal
Genitourinary
Musculoskeletal
Neurologic
Psychiatric
Allergic/immunologic/lymphatic
Rheumatologic
Endocrine

situations, when information gathering is necessarily truncated by multiple admissions and other stresses on the medical system itself, and by limitations in the patient's own recollection and knowledge. At least three strategies can be used to avoid these pitfalls:

1. Obtain the information in multiple settings.
2. Make use of a team approach—often the medical student, physician's assistant, or members of the nursing staff will extract key information that is missed by other caregivers.
3. When available and appropriate, always use prior medical records and family sources to supplement the patient's memory.

At the same time, the verbal presentation of a comprehensive ROS too often becomes a time sink. Students and house officers often give an exhaustive and exhausting recitation of positives and negatives. *Although essential to the written history, this type of extra information causes the oral presentation to bog down.*

The most condensed form of presentation is simply a statement that the "Review of systems is positive for . . . " followed by the relevant information. Be mindful of situations in which the ROS is "grossly positive." Furthermore, if truly relevant to the CC, the pertinent positives or negatives might be given in the HPI. From the example above, additional information would help frame the context of the abdominal pain: *Mrs. Jones denies any melena, hematochezia, weight loss, or loss of appetite.*

In the example of a 50-year-old patient who presents with documented fevers up to 101.7°F and night sweats for a month, the differential diagnosis centers importantly on infection (e.g., HIV, bacterial endocarditis, tuberculosis), and cancer (especially lymphoma). A concise ROS could be:

> *She reports a 10-pound weight loss over the past month, but denies any rashes, sore throat, cough, or hemoptysis.*

However, again, it may be preferable to include these key positives and negatives in the HPI.

> Your attendings may have strong preferences about how they like the ROS presented, and it is best to clarify these early. You will need to develop and use judgment in selecting which information is relevant. It is always advisable to add carefully selected negatives and positives that bear directly on diagnoses you are considering.

Similarly, the family history can be an aspect of the presentation that gets bogged down with excessive detail or weakened by inadequate history taking. For example, in a patient admitted with cholecystitis, relaying that the patient's parents had asthma is not important. In a 65-year-old man admitted with chest pain, knowing that his father had an MI when he was 50 years old is extremely helpful. Furthermore, sometimes valuable clues may be "buried" and emerge only after some detective work.

EXAMPLE

A 36-year-old woman with a history of anxiety is admitted for lightheadedness and palpitations. She had a similar episode three years ago, and recalls similar instances as a teenager. She denies frank syncope, and her episodes have never been associated with chest pain. She is on no medications, and aside from the symptoms reported in the HPI, her ROS is unremarkable. Her 12-lead electrocardiogram raises concern for a prolonged QT interval (corrected QTc 470 ms). The patient denies any history of arrhythmia or any coronary artery disease. Later, it is discovered that her sister died from drowning while swimming in a lake, and her paternal uncle died from sudden infant death syndrome. Given this newly revealed aspect of the history, there was enhanced suspicion for sudden death due to arrhythmia. Genotyping was performed, and she was found to have a mutation in the KCNQ1 locus, which has been isolated to chromosome 11, responsible for a common type of hereditary long QT syndrome (Figure 1.1). Her younger siblings, both of whom were asymptomatic, agreed to genetic screening; one sibling was found to be positive for the mutation as well. The patient was given a betablocker and referred to a cardiologist and genetic counselor.

Normal QT (rate corrected QT interval = 395 ms; normal ≤440 ms)

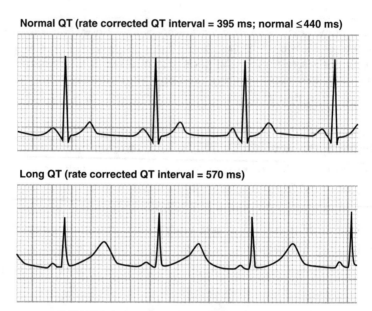

Long QT (rate corrected QT interval = 570 ms)

FIGURE 1.1   Normal and long QT intervals.

In this example, detailed history taking helped uncover the diagnosis of a subtle but life-threatening cardiac electrophysiologic syndrome. The family history prompted genetic testing for one of the more common inherited causes of sudden cardiac arrest. (Obviously, genetic screening is inappropriate for every patient who presents with palpitations and light-headedness. The long-term management of patients such as this, as well as for patients who have the genetic mutation but who are asymptomatic, is a subject of much debate.)

Past Medical History

A past medical history (PMH) must be presented in full as part of the admission note. Based on the attending's preferences and specialty, it may be thematically subgrouped into past medical, past surgical, past psychiatric, past obstetric, and so on. At times, as with the examples above of coronary artery disease and diabetes mellitus, details of the past history are presented in the HPI because of their immediate relevance to these two major disease processes. What if the patient is being admitted for a problem (e.g., a tibial fracture after being hit by a bicycle) that is not apparently related to coronary disease or diabetes? In such cases, the details of these two problems could be presented separately in the PMH section. However, because of the multisystem nature of conditions such as diabetes mellitus, which may affect therapy, if not diagnosis, on rounds one might present the past medical history succinctly by saying "the patient's past medical history is notable for asymptomatic coronary artery disease, status post angioplasty of the left anterior descending artery two years ago, and for stable type 2 diabetes mellitus, which is diet-controlled." In the write-up, appropriate details can be provided.

Finally, uncovering the past medical history may be challenging, especially if the patient is a "poor historian" because of age, complicated management, stress, effects of a chronic or acute process on memory, and if reliable medical records are incomplete or unavailable. In some cases, a patient's medications may be helpful (see below). As an example, if the patient is known to be on metformin and glipizide, the diagnosis of diabetes mellitus is virtually assured. On the other hand, finding that the patient is on digoxin does not necessarily mean that he or she has heart failure or an atrial arrhythmia—often, patients are still on medications prescribed years ago for a remote or even misdiagnosed problem, or when "archaic" prescriptions are never discontinued. A certain amount of imaginative detective work may be required with calls to physicians named on prescriptions, the pharmacies, and of course, family members with instructions to "bring in all the pill bottles" as discussed further below.

Medication Profile

The importance of a complete medication history cannot be overemphasized. The medication profile should include both current and, where possible to document, prior medications and adverse medication reactions. This category includes two distinct features that are very different but often confused, especially by patients: (1) allergies and (2) side effects and intolerances. Furthermore, a variety of sources suggest that at least 10–20% of Americans use herbal or other supplemental medications, and most often do not report this use to their medical practitioners.

A common and important error is to give an incomplete rendering of a patient's drug history or current medication profile. For example, a typical statement might be:

> *Mr. Kramer is on the following medications: (1) atorvastatin 20 mg, once a day; (2) hydrochlorothiazide 25 mg, once a day; (3) aspirin 81 mg, once a day; (4) metoprolol succinate 50 mg, once a day; and (5) zolpidem, 10 mg, at night, as needed.*

What is missing from this summary?

Adherence/Compliance

Is Mr. Kramer actually taking the medications as prescribed? A consistent finding in medical surveys is the low level of adherence with prescribed medications. Just because a patient relates "being on" certain medications is no guarantee that the medications are actually being *taken as prescribed, or taken at all.* Adherence rates as low as 43–78% have been reported for patients taking medications prescribed for chronic conditions. Such nonadherence can have major consequences during a hospital admission, as the patient is usually guaranteed to receive those medications *as prescribed* rather than the dosages actually taken at home. For example, in cases such as "treatment-resistant" hypertension, precipitous falls in blood pressure may occur upon exposure to the assumed doses of antihypertensives.

Many reasons for nonadherence are identifiable (Exhibit 1.3), including inability of the patient to afford the medication; unreported intolerance or side effects (not actual allergies) of the medication (e.g., headache, nausea, diarrhea), confusion about the indication for the medication, lack of belief in the therapy, contradictory inputs from multiple caregivers, psychiatric syndromes, and multidose regimens.

Even among professional caregivers, compliance rates are rather low. One study of physicians and nurses by Rhonda Corda, M.P.H., and her colleagues at New York Medical College (2000) revealed that only about 80% of respondents reported taking medications properly

EXHIBIT 1.3   Major Predictors of Poor Adherence to Medication

Presence of psychological problems, particularly depression
Presence of cognitive impairment
Treatment of asymptomatic disease
Inadequate follow-up or discharge planning
Side effects of medication
Patient's lack of belief in benefit of treatment
Patient's lack of insight into the illness
Poor provider–patient relationship
Presence of barriers to care or medication
Missed appointments
Complexity of treatment
Cost of medication, copayment, or both

Source: Adapted from Osterberg L, Blaschke T. Adherence to medication. N Engl J Med. 2005;353:487–497.

80% or more of the time. As the authors noted, expecting patients to exceed their physicians in compliance with medications is unlikely.

> As a rule, always assume that one or more medications are not being taken as prescribed and that the patient may be taking others (self-prescribed, such as herbals and other supplements) not reported initially.

An important and probably underreported source of medication errors is the tendency to automatically transcribe in admission orders the same medications that a patient reported to be taking at home or on transfer in the identical doses. A related common pitfall is to use the discharge medications from a prior hospitalization list as a surrogate for a current medication profile because that list reflects medications the patient was *reliably receiving and taking* while hospitalized. This "reflex" can have a number of serious and even fatal consequences. The admission itself may be due to a medication allergy or intolerance. Reordering the same panel of medications may therefore inadvertently perpetuate the disease process that caused the admission. As such, *medication reconciliation* is absolutely critical to patient care. This term (see Exhibit 1.4) refers to the interactive multistage process of identifying and cross-checking the most accurate, updated

---

EXHIBIT 1.4   The Four Steps of Medication Reconciliation

Step 1: Obtain and document the most complete and accurate list possible for all current medications.

Step 2: Compare the "home medications" listed with any new orders, to reconcile discrepancies.

Step 3: Update the list as orders change during the clinic/office visit or hospital stay and make necessary and appropriate medication changes based on the patient's clinical condition.

Step 4: Communicate the updated list to the next provider of service and to the patient when the patient is transferred to another setting, service, practitioner, or level of care within or outside the organization.

---

list of all medications your patient is taking, including name, dosage, frequency, and route, and then using this list to provide correct medications for the patient anywhere within the health care system.

EXAMPLE

45-year-old woman with poorly controlled insulin-dependent diabetes mellitus, cryptogenic cirrhosis, and a history of GI bleeding in the past secondary to esophageal varices, was admitted to the hospital from liver clinic due to a markedly elevated plasma glucose of 682 mg/dL. The admitting team restarted her home insulin regimen, as listed from her last clinic note, written two months ago. Shortly afterward, she was found unresponsive, with a blood glucose reading of 21 mg/dL. She received 1 ampule dextrose 50% in water and was intubated for airway protection given that her mental status did not improve with the intravenous glucose bolus.

After anesthesia induction, she became hypotensive with systolic blood pressures in the range 70 to 80 mmHg, which did not respond to intravenous fluids. She was started on phenylephrine and then norepinephrine and her blood pressure normalized. This episode was also associated with elevation of cardiac biomarkers—her troponin I was elevated to 2.61 ng/mL, and a transthoracic echo revealed an ejection fraction of 15% with inferior wall akinesis and severely decreased left ventricular systolic function. Of note, an echocardiogram performed three months prior as part of a liver transplant workup showed a normal ejection fraction at 60% with normal right and left ventricular systolic function.

Subsequent history revealed that the patient was extremely non-compliant with her home insulin regimen, and the dose listed in the chart was much higher than what she was actually taking. At outpatient follow-up one month later, his left ventricular ejection fraction had returned to normal as assessed by echocardiography.

Lack of medication reconciliation can have serious and even life-threatening effects and accounts for an estimated 50% of all medication errors and up to 20% of adverse drug events in the hospital setting. In the example above, failure to document the actual dose of insulin led to a series of life-threatening complications.

In the case of Mr. Kramer, mentioned earlier, a preferable statement would be:

> *Mr. Kramer reports taking the following medications prescribed by his PCP at Longview Creek: [Give meds]. Of note, he says that he has missed two weeks of these pills because he ran out of his prescriptions, [or] He says he has been compliant with these pills and took the last doses of all of them yesterday.*

Other consequences of reflex prescribing include giving medications that may interfere with imminent surgical procedures (e.g., warfarin) and continuing medications that interact with one or more drugs that are being added to the current regimen without consideration of dose modification. Digitalis toxicity, including potentially serious brady- or tachyarrhythmias, may ensue.

EXAMPLE

An 81-year-old man presented to the emergency department complaining of 6 weeks of fatigue, malaise, and loss of appetite. He denied fever, night sweats, abdominal discomfort, or change of mental status. Three weeks earlier he had been evaluated for an episode of syncope at another hospital, where he was found to be in atrial fibrillation with a rapid ventricular response at approximately 150 beats per minute. He was treated with intravenous heparin and started on 5 mg of warfarin in anticipation of chemical cardioversion with amiodarone. After a 300 mg IV amiodarone bolus with subsequent infusion over 18 hours, he converted to sinus rhythm. Heparin was discontinued once he was therapeutically anticoagulated with warfarin. He was then started on digoxin 0.125 mg daily. On discharge, he was prescribed oral amiodarone, digoxin, and warfarin and instructed to follow up with his primary care physician. He returned shortly afterward with the symptoms noted above—his trough serum digoxin level was 5.6 ng/mL, far in excess of the conservative therapeutic range (preferably <1.0 ng/mL).

In this case, the seemingly nonspecific complaints of an elderly man turn out to be symptoms of a life-threatening iatrogenic problem: digitalis toxicity. Digoxin interacts with numerous commonly prescribed drugs, especially those taken by patients with heart failure, for which digoxin is often prescribed (thiazide and "loop" diuretics, calcium-channel blockers, and antiarrhythmics). Amiodarone increases the steady-state concentration of digitalis and may cause a twofold increase in the serum digoxin level. As such, maintenance doses of digoxin should be reduced by 50% in those also taking amiodarone.

This case also raises another important issue: the potential overuse of drugs without documented indications. Digoxin has a narrow therapeutic margin and is mainly indicated in chronic symptomatic systolic heart failure and as an adjunct to maintaining a controlled ventricular response in atrial fibrillation (see Chapter 8). Further, the use of digoxin to prevent atrial fibrillation has not been documented. In retrospect, its use in this case, where the patient was discharged in sinus rhythm without heart failure, lacked compelling justification.

> *Three Important Rx Rules:*
>
> - *Never* reflexively put patients on the same medications they report taking without critically reviewing each prescription and the dosage/ formulation with the patient or responsible caretaker.
> - *Always* look for potential drug interactions between current and newly prescribed medications, as well as appropriate adjustments for age and other factors that may affect volume of distribution and clearance.
> - *Always* question the indication for a given drug and critically assess the published evidence for efficacy in patients with characteristics similar to those in the patient who you are treating.

Over and Under the Counter

As mentioned above, an important but often overlooked aspect of the medication history is documentation of nonformulary medications and supplements. This topic has received increased attention in the medical and popular press recently, with the important finding that substantial numbers of patients in the United States and other countries take a variety of complementary and alternative medications and utilize a wide range of interventions outside the sphere of traditional medical practice. This phenomenon is, of course, independent of the "recreational" use of illegal substances, which is also widespread and an essential part of the medical history.

EXAMPLE

You are seeing a 44-year-old man with HIV infection in your hospital clinic for routine follow-up. He was diagnosed initially 5 years ago, and last saw his infectious disease physician 6 weeks ago. He has always been asymptomatic, and at last check his CD4 count was 500 per cubic millimeter and his viral load was undetectable (<50 copies per milliliter). He has been compliant with his HIV regimen: a protease inhibitor (lopinavir–ritonovir, 800 and 200 mg once daily as a fixed-dose combination), and two nucleoside reverse-transcriptase inhibitors (zidovudine–lamivudine, 300 and 150 mg, twice daily as a fixed-dose combination). He reports having difficulty with his finances and reports feeling depressed, with fatigue and loss of interest in his favorite pastimes of gardening and yoga. You initiate a discussion of antidepressant medications (checking for drug–drug interactions). He then reveals that he started taking St. John's wort (*Hypericum perfora-tum*) one month ago at the recommendation of a friend. You promptly page his infectious disease physician for consultation.

Comment: This vignette is important because it illustrates how elucidating a "hidden history"—in this case, taking St. John's wort—averted potentially life-threatening complications. This herbal supplement can have major interactions with HIV treatment (lowering serum concentrations) along with many other commonly prescribed medications [e.g., warfarin (reduced effect), paroxetine (grogginess and lethargy), oral contraceptives (reduced efficacy), and cyclosporine (reduced levels)]. Another example is provided by garlic (*Allium sativum*) supplements, which may reduce the level of certain protease inhibitors, such as saquinivar, and enhance the effects of antiplatelet agents and of warfarin. Certain herbal medications may also affect anesthetic management.

Exhibit 1.5 is a more comprehensive list of substances considered as medications that goes well beyond prescribed and nonprescribed pharmacy-type agents (e.g., vaccines, radioactive preparations, blood derivatives, respiratory therapy-related agents, and a variety of others).

ADVERSE EFFECTS

Take care not to confuse true medication *allergies* (i.e., immunologically mediated effects such as rash, laryngospasm, bronchospasm, angioedema, pruritis, and urticaria) with *medication intolerance* or other nonimmunological side effects (e.g., nausea, weakness, diarrhea, headache, dizziness). Furthermore, not infrequently, patients mistake an allergy for a drug's pronounced desired effect (e.g., bradycardia with beta-blockers, nausea with disulfuram). In the latter

EXHIBIT 1.5   What Is a Medication?

Prescription medications
Sample medications
Vitamins
Nutraceuticals (e.g., dietary supplements and herbal products)
Over-the-counter (nonprescription) drugs (e.g., common allergy and cold
   formulations)
Vaccines
Diagnostic and contrast agents
Radioactive medications (e.g., radioactive iodine for hyperthyroidism)
Respiratory therapy-related medications
Parenteral nutrition
Blood derivatives
Intravenous solutions (plain or with additives)
Any other product designated as a drug by the U.S. Food and Drug Administration

Note: This official list, based on the Joint Commission, does not include biologically active chemicals that you might have added as other candidate "drugs," including recreational/illicit substances, caffeinated drinks, and nicotine-containing tobacco products. Is exercise a medication? What about certain types of light exposure? What else is missing from this list?

example, the fact that an adverse effect is not a true allergy does not mean that it cannot be life-threatening. Consider hypotension and bradycardia due to blood pressure medications, which may induce syncope, with disastrous consequences. Another class of examples includes the *proarrhythmic effects* of drugs used to treat arrhythmias (e.g., flecainide, propafenone). Such drugs may actually cause or promote life-threatening electrical instability associated with cardiac arrest and sudden death (N Engl J Med. 1989;321:406–412).

Always review allergies and intolerances, as several medications that are routinely (and automatically) prescribed on standardized order sets on hospital admission (e.g., acetaminophen, diphenhydramine, promethazine, prochlorperazine, morphine sulfate) may cause allergies or side effects. More often than not, some of the allergies reported are wholly incorrect, and preclude the use of that agent in favor of one that may be more expensive or less effective.

For example, in patients following acute myocardial infarction, aspirin decreases risk for recurrent infarction and for death. However, a reported allergy to aspirin may preclude providers from administering this medication when in truth the "allergy" is simply an instance of gastrointestinal upset. True allergies to aspirin do occur but are relatively rare.

> [I]t's easy to write prescriptions, but difficult to come to an understanding with people.
> —FRANZ KAFKA (1883–1924), *Country Doctor*

Attending's Perspective on Presentations:
Freeze-Framing Technique

The discussion above on presenting cases, directed primarily at students and house officers, is aimed at improving their communication skills vis-à-vis each other and their attendings. However, attendings have an added challenge beyond deciphering often overly long and less than optimally organized presentations. They not only need to assimilate and integrate the data and vet its reliability but also need to interrupt the presentation at selected points for clarification and teaching purposes. Individual preferences will guide whether one favors letting a presentation run its course or whether interruptions are helpful. The authors favor the latter, especially during walking or sitting-down teaching rounds. One particularly useful strategy for attendings (and residents) is to *freeze* the presentation at key stages and ask what members of the team are thinking. This procedure will not only help prevent junior colleagues from having mental "walkabouts," but is also essential for developing skills in actively processing information and developing differential diagnosis skills.

For example, you are listening to a presentation that begins:

> *Janice Ripley is a 37-year-old woman previously well who presents to our medical center for the first time, complaining of "feeling short of breath" for 1 week.*

A dramatic device for teaching, and one that may help elucidate the cause of this patient's dyspnea, is to stop the presentation abruptly and ask: What is the differential diagnosis of dyspnea in a 37-year-old woman given no other information? The ensuing discussion, which can be brief, would encompass (1) *pulmonary* (thromboembolic syndromes, obstructive disease, restrictive disease due, for example, to infection, metastatic cancer or pleural effusion with lung compression, pneumothorax, etc.), (2) *cardiac* (heart failure or an anginal equivalent), (3) *metabolic* (anemia, or acidosis with Kussmaul respiration), and (4) *psychogenic* (anxiety) etiologies.

As the case develops, you can interrupt again to ask how the new information helps focus on one or more of the initial broad range of possibilities or what was not mentioned that may be relevant (e.g., recent travel with prolonged sitting on a plane, or intake of oral contraceptives, both of which would increase the pretest probability of thromboembolic disease). No prescription exists or should exist for how many times per diem a presentation should be freeze-framed or what the questions should be. Indeed, scores of possibilities exist as the attending becomes a role model of active listening and clinical hypothesis generation and testing.

Overall, it is helpful to point out, up front, what you expect from student presentations, and be aware that it is likely to differ from others' preferences. Students will always adopt their own styles and preferences as they become more senior, and their preferred method of hearing and giving presentations may be biased toward what they learn early on—in both positive and negative ways.

The term *teachable moment* has entered politics as well as medicine and other disciplines. The authors declare their bias/opinion here that the term, like most buzzwords, has lost whatever meaning it may originally have had. In medicine, all "moments" are potentially teachable, constrained only by time and priorities. Selecting the obvious ones weights them unduly and may draw attention away from the equally important but less apparent "clinical pearls."

MINI-SUMMARY

- Patient history write-ups and oral summaries (narratives) are often marred by being disorganized and too lengthy.
- Trim your written ROS to include only pertinent positives and negatives in oral presentations.

- Medication history is often incomplete with respect to accuracy, adherence, dosage, and allergies/intolerances. These lapses can cause disastrous consequences.
- Medication lists need to be reconciled (updated) every time a patient is seen as an in- or outpatient and made available to all health care providers.

CHAPTER 2

REEXAMINING THE PHYSICAL EXAM

Then he felt her pulse. There was a strong stroke and a weak one, like a sound and its echo. That was supposed to betoken the end.
                                    —D.H. LAWRENCE (1885–1930), *Sons and Lovers*

Our senses as diagnostic aids have been almost completely replaced by laboratory instruments and the consequences may sometimes be disastrous.
                                    —LOUIS K. DIAMOND, M.D. (1902–1999)

Dr. Louis Diamond, a clinical giant and a pioneer in the field of pediatric hematology, was entirely on target with his warning about the attrition of physical diagnostic skills over the past decades. Clinicians have come to overrely on "definitive" imaging studies for diagnoses. Multiple studies, including computed tomography (CT) scans, magnetic resonance imaging (MRI), and ultrasonography (Figure 2.1), reveal information beyond the sensitivity of human observers and may confirm and quantify findings. Such studies are invaluable triumphs of modern biotechnology.

Becoming a Consummate Clinician: What Every Student, House Officer, and Hospital Practitioner Needs to Know, First Edition.
Ary L. Goldberger and Zachary D. Goldberger.

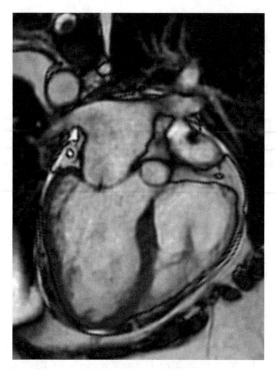

FIGURE 2.1   A magnetic resonance imaging study of a heart with hypertrophic cardiomyopathy. Courtesy of Hussein Rayatzadeh, M.D.

Conversely, to the degree that imaging studies dull perceptive skills, clinicians and students need to be very cautious. A careful physical exam remains a mainstay of clinical diagnosis and management. Cross-checking every aspect of the exam by some imaging or other test is both costly and infeasible. In addition, some studies, such as x-rays and computerized tomographic (CT) scans, may subject patients to unnecessary radiation exposure. Other tests, such as tissue biopsies, carry obvious risks. Furthermore, imaging studies have important diagnostic limitations with respect to sensitivity and specificity. Adding to their expense and risk, the more tests you order, the more you are likely to generate false positives or otherwise misleading findings. On the other hand, failure to recognize the limited sensitivity of a test may result in missed diagnoses.

The physical exam is therefore not only vital but should be repeated as often as needed. For example, the presence of a new murmur after a myocardial infarction may herald a potentially catastrophic condition, such as a ventricular septal defect, acute mitral regurgitation from papillary muscle rupture, or left ventricular free wall rupture. But above all, the "laying on of hands" in a thoughtful and compassionate way is an essential part of the unique connection between clinician and patient. As Sir William Osler advised:

> Remember . . . that every patient upon whom you wait will examine you critically and form an estimate of you by the way in which you conduct yourself at the bedside. Skill and nicety in manipulation, in the simple act of feeling the pulse or in the performance of any minor operation will do more towards establishing confidence in you, than a string of Diplomas, or the reputation of extensive hospital experience.

A major theme is that examining a patient is a form of focused questioning or *hypothesis testing*, a special type of active, iterative, and interrogatory process shaped by the patient's presenting complaint and history. This notion of a dynamic rather than a passive exam is critically important because it underscores the necessity to "look, listen, and feel *for* findings," not just *at* them. Many important findings do not jump out at you; you have to hunt for them. Although some findings are obvious (e.g., marked scleral icterus, severe clubbing of the fingers and toes), most are not. For example, you will almost certainly never notice Cheyne–Stokes breathing (in heart failure or stroke) or pulsus paradoxus (in pericardial tamponade or severe obstructive lung disease) unless you look for them, as illustrated further below. In doing so, you are testing, asking directing questions and sometimes posing actual hypotheses, referred to more informally as hunches. ("I am testing the hypothesis that this patient has physical findings consistent with hyperthyroidism.")

PHYSICAL EXAM AND HYPOTHESIS TESTING

The physical exam is often taught with an emphasis on "observational findings" from regional components [head, eyes, ears, nose, and throat, neck, thoracic (chest, heart), abdominal, etc.]. In addition, students should conceptualize the exam not only in terms of these component (regional) parts, but of more systemic (integrated) features and be guided by active questioning and hypothesis testing, not just passive observation. For example, in examining the thyroid gland area, the key parameters (by inspection and palpation at baseline and during swallowing) are its estimated size, consistency, tenderness, and presence of nodularity/masses. The most basic (ground level) questions might be: Does the patient have a normal-feeling gland or enlarged thyroid (goiter), the latter most consistent with hyperthyroidism? Is there evidence of nodularity (single or multiple) or other masses? Is the thyroid area tender, consistent with thyroiditis? The more advanced the examiner, the more refined the questions, hypotheses, and exam techniques will be. (See Chapter 11 and the "nautilus shell" learning approach.)

From a systemic point of view, informed by the patient's history, you may also be testing hypotheses that require complex integration and coordination of multiple components of the exam. For example, if your guess (hypothesis) is that your patient has hyperthyroidism, you will be addressing a number of specific questions: Is there resting tachycardia or a fast irregular rhythm, suggesting atrial fibrillation? Is there a fine resting tremor of the hands? Noticeable sweatiness? Is there lid-lag or a characteristic stare? Is there frank proptosis (exophthalmos), specifically suggesting Graves' disease as the etiology of the hyperthyroidism? Is there a thyroid bruit? Muscle weakness consistent with myopathy? A nonpitting type of indurated, pretibial edema (confusingly called pretibial myxedema)? Cardiovascular findings consistent with high-output heart failure? Integration of findings also helps increase certainty about disease status. For example, a borderline prominent thyroid gland in the presence of a constellation of several other findings typical of hyperthyroidism increases the probability that an apparently enlarged gland is abnormally hyperactive.

The concept of the physical exam as an integrated dynamic set of observations, directed questions, and hypothesis testing can help trainees think creatively and physiologically. Consider the cardiac exam. Traditionally, the centerpiece, literally and figuratively, is auscultation of the heart. However, by the time that experienced cardiologists apply their stethoscopes to the chest, they may have "upregulated" their sensory apparatus by looking for and finding other clues. For example, low-amplitude carotid pulses with delayed upstrokes strongly suggest advanced aortic stenosis. Hearing bilateral bruits over the carotids raises the differential diagnosis of local stenosis vs. a transmitted murmur. Testing to see if the point of maximal impulse is sustained further supports a pressure load. In the absence of hypertension (the most common cause of a pressure load on the left ventricle), the probability of critical aortic stenosis is raised even further in the presence of these findings, well in advance of auscultation. With advanced aortic insufficiency (regurgitation), cardiac auscultation may also be "anticlimactic" since you will probably make or suspect a diagnosis based on systolic hypertension with a widened pulse pressure and bounding pulses.

A second major theme of this chapter is that *the physical examination can be viewed as a coordinated series of lab tests, each component of which has its own limitations in sensitivity, specificity, and predictive values.* Failure to appreciate the elements of a physical exam as the equivalent of a set of lab tests may lead to diagnostic errors, including both oversights (false negatives) and overcalls (false positives). For example, according to McGee's textbook (see the Bibliography), the absence of a goiter by palpation or inspection has a sensitivity (versus ultrasound measures or surgical weight as the "gold standards") of only 5 to 57% and a specificity of only 0 to 26%. In contrast, the presence of a goiter by palpation has a higher reported sensitivity (between 43 and 82%) and specificity between 88 and 100%. These figures are of note for at least two reasons: (1) they indicate the large disparity from one study to another in assessing medical diagnostics, and (2) they suggest that clinicians are much more likely to underestimate than to overestimate the presence of an enlarged thyroid.

Recognizing and quantifying the imprecision of a physical finding does not detract at all from the scientific nature of the exam; rather, it puts the exam on a firmer scientific basis so that the positive and negative findings can be assessed more objectively and quantitatively. Also, studies that analyze the exam critically may motivate innovative diagnostic modalities or maneuvers that enhance the accuracy of the physical exam. The ability of students to correlate their physical findings with objective imaging studies (ultrasound exams, cardiac catheterizations, MRI and CT scans, or direct tissue studies from biopsies or the operating room) provides an invaluable way of honing examination skills.

A number of superb texts detail the uses and limitations of the physical exam; some are cited in the Bibliography, including the *JAMA* evidence-based clinical diagnosis text, *The Rational Clinical Examination*, edited by Dr. David Simel and Dr. Drummond Rennie and Dr. Steven McGee's book, *Evidence-Based Physical Diagnosis*. The purpose here is to emphasize essential aspects of the exam that are often performed incompletely or described incorrectly in oral and written presentations.

Worth reemphasizing is the importance of examining patients with direct visualization and palpation, not through the gown, which can mask findings (e.g., skin lesions), decrease tactile sensitivity, and lead to false-positive findings (e.g., spurious "rales").

GENERAL APPEARANCE

The summary of the physical exam must always begin with a brief sentence or two describing the general appearance of the patient. This first element in the physical examination places the entire case in context. Here are some examples:

Case 1. Mr. Jones is a young adult man in no apparent distress, asking when he can be discharged.

Case 2. Ms. Smith is a middle-aged woman complaining of severe chest pain and sweating profusely.

Case 3. Ms. Roberts is a very pale elderly woman intubated and sedated, making intermittent groaning sounds.

The general appearance of the patient is a key aspect of the physical examination and should always be described in written and oral presentations, no matter how abbreviated. This description will guide the pace of the remainder of the evaluation (e.g., if the patient has unexplainable mental status changes and slurred speech or is in extreme pain). This assessment is one of the facets that distinguish students from residents from seasoned attendings: The ability to sense how sick your patient may be is not only the initial part but also one of the most valuable aspects of the physical exam.

REVITALIZING THE VITAL SIGNS

Perhaps the most important short-changed features of an exam are appropriately termed the *vital signs*. However, despite their centrality in the exam, even the definition of what constitutes the vital signs is subject to describer variability and some controversy. Universally, clinicians include a minimum of four measurements in the vital signs: body temperature, heart rate, respiration, and blood pressure. The patient's perception of pain is sometimes included. Additionally, the authors concur with those who add height (may be self-reported by the patient) and weight (should always be measured), and, if indicated, noninvasive oxygen blood content (pulse oximetry). The latter is usually obtained at the bedside by a probe placed on the earlobe or finger and expressed as SpO_2. This is not SaO_2, or true arterial saturation, which is not available unless you have access to blood from an indwelling arterial catheter in an intensive care unit (ICU).

What is rarely, if ever, discussed on rounds is how devices such as oximetry probes are actually designed to work. Although most physicians are not engineers, a general knowledge of the equipment we use is interesting and helpful in understanding the artifacts and limitations of these devices.

> Given our reliance on devices and laboratory measurements, it is extremely helpful to understand the "physiology" of these devices and instruments—how they function correctly. In addition, it is important to know something about their "pathophysiology"—how they can malfunction, or produce spurious results.

The Pulse Oximeter This widely used device (Figure 2.2) measures the percentage of hemoglobin in arterial blood, which is saturated with oxygen, or the SpO_2 (as well as the heart rate). Pulse oximeters contain a probe with a pair of diodes that emit light with two discrete wavelengths: red (~650 nm, which is visible when the oximeter is turned on) and infrared (~900 nm, which cannot be seen). Pulse oximeters direct light beams of these wavelengths through a translucent site on the body (typically, a finger, toe, or earlobe) onto a photodetector placed on the opposite side of the anatomical site.

Well-oxygenated blood absorbs most of the infrared light transmitted through the oximeter and allows more of the red light to pass through. Conversely, deoxygenated (reduced) hemoglobin, which is darker in color, absorbs more of the red-wavelength light and allows more infrared light to pass through to the detector. The oxyhemoglobin/deoxyhemoglobin ratio can then be calculated from the ratio of the absorption of the red and infrared light by a microprocessor in the device. This ratio is compared against empirically derived values which correspond to given oxygen saturation levels. Of note, the oxygen content in tissues that do not generate pulsatile flow (e.g., muscle, fat, bone, venous blood) is not measured.

Knowing the basic "physiology" of how a pulse oximeter works under normal circumstances enables one to understand the conditions under which the device may malfunction or the readings be unreliable—the device "pathophysiology." For example, SpO_2 by pulse oximetry can be (1) spuriously high with carbon monoxide poisoning since the devices do not distinguish between oxyhemoglobin and carboxyhemoglobin, or (2) spuriously low (e.g., in the rare case of methemoglobinemia or in the presence of dark nail polish that may block light transmission). Physiological conditions that cause spuriously low readings include low-output states (e.g., cardiogenic or hypovolemic shock), since both are associated with decreased amplitude of arterial pulsations.

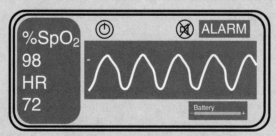

FIGURE 2.2 A pulse oximeter.

EXAMPLE

A 65-year-old man was brought to the emergency department after his friends found him to be confused and dysarthric, lying on the floor of his mobile home. He was unable to provide a clear history due to his mental status. His initial vital signs revealed a temperature of 38.5°C, heart rate 112 bpm, BP 80/65 mmHg, resting heart rate 25/min, and SpO$_2$ 96% on ambient air. His Glasgow Coma score was 12. He had an elevated creatinine kinase at 14,359 IU/L. His chest x-ray was suggestive of a possible small left lower lobe infiltrate. A urine and serum toxicology screen was negative. Blood and urine cultures were negative. He was treated empirically with antibiotics for a presumed pneumonia. Despite an extensive workup for mental status changes including a brain MRI, EEG, and a lumbar puncture, a diagnosis was not found. After a seven-day admission, his mental status improved, and further history was obtained. He recalled turning on his gas heating for the first time since the spring. A carboxyhemoglobin level was found to be 10%. He was discharged, and his heater was turned off and repaired.

Comment: Carbon monoxide (CO) poisoning can cause a myriad of clinical symptoms, ranging from mild nausea to severe central nervous system (CNS) toxicity and even death. Although hyperbaric oxygen therapy is sometimes used in cases of acute poisoning, symptoms due to chronic exposure to relatively low levels of carbon monoxide—as in the case of this patient—usually resolve after removal from the exposure. Pulse oximetry was normal and remained normal during admission. A CO oximeter is needed to determine carboxyhemoglobin levels. A standard pulse oximeter will *not* detect CO poisoning because the carboxyhemoglobin will be misdetected as normal hemoglobin.

Every admission exam should enumerate vital sign measures and specify which ones are not available. And although you may not be the one taking the initial vital signs (usually performed at first in the emergency department, or by another member of the health care team in the inpatient or outpatient setting), make every effort to confirm them yourself. For example, it may be literally life-saving if you notice a 30-mmHg drop in systolic blood pressure compared to a reading recorded as normal 1 hour prior.

You should train yourself to avoid the following lapses, both minor and major:

- Failing to be complete—leaving out one or more of the vital signs or not describing them fully is surprisingly common.
- Failing to give appropriate units in the write-up. The exam should be considered a unique type of scientific observational study ($n = 1$). Scientific biomedical measurements most often are given in specified units; exceptions include special cases such as the inspiratory/expiratory ratio, where the units cancel out.
- For heights and weights, either the metric or English systems can be used. However, you should be internally consistent so that you are not listing someone as 5 feet 8 inches and 70 kg. Even more aggravating to your attendings is the practice of recording weight in kilograms one day and switching to pounds the next. Three major sources of variability in this essential vital sign are: (1) measurement at different times of the day (before and after meals or medications such as diuretics), (2) the use of different scales, and (3) different amounts of clothing being worn by the patient.

Note that SpO_2 is measured as a percentage (%).

ADDITIONAL LAPSES IN REPORTING THE VITAL SIGNS

Aside from not assigning proper units to the vital signs, a much more serious source of error is in actually mismeasuring or representing them incompletely. Considering that the vital signs are the most accessible and objective of physical findings, this common flaw is surprising and calls into question apparently less objective and more subtle measurements that follow. Being more precise and scientific in how you report and expect the vital signs to be reported will raise the bar on your other clinical communications. Rigor breeds rigor.

For heart rate, it is appropriate to add a tag line indicating the cadence of the heartbeat: whether it is regular, grossly irregular, or intermittently irregular. Stating "normal sinus rhythm" or "regular sinus rhythm" in the physical is not appropriate, however, since sinus rhythm is a finding based on an electrocardiogram (ECG), not on a physical exam. For example, the heart rate could be 75 beats per minute and regular with atrial flutter and 4:1 atrioventricular (AV) conduction rather than with sinus rhythm. [A very canny observer in the latter case may note flutter waves in the jugular venous pressure (JVP) displacements in the neck.] Furthermore, it is impossible from the physical exam alone to detect the presence of an ectopic atrial rhythm at a physiologic rate.

In describing the cardiac rhythm, we discourage use of the widely used term *irregularly irregular* because it has come to connote specifically atrial fibrillation. Thus, if you say that the pulse is irregularly irregular, you will imply to most observers a diagnosis of atrial fibrillation. However, on exam at four common distinct rhythms—sinus rhythm with frequent atrial or ventricular premature beats, wandering atrial pacemaker/multifocal atrial tachycardia, atrial flutter with variable AV conduction, and atrial fibrillation—all feel "irregularly irregular." The two former rhythms are not indications of anticoagulation, whereas atrial fibrillation usually is. Other rhythms may cause considerable variability in heart rate as well. Finally, respiratory sinus arrhythmia—the phasic increase and decrease in heart rate due to alterations in vagal tone as a result of respiration—may cause the pulse to be variable over a period of seconds (Chapter 9).

Thus, these terminological suggestions are not meant as fussy distinctions without differences. Also, the use of "irregularly irregular" implies the presence of a companion set of rhythms that are "regularly irregular." But the latter term would be considered baffling by most of your colleagues and is not used clinically. (Some advocate using this term for AV Wenckebach with its periodic cycles—we would advise reporting that the pulse was variable in a possibly periodic way.)

From an interpretive point of view, failure to appreciate the importance of a resting tachycardia can also lead to missed or belated diagnoses. The usual resting heart rate ("normal sinus rhythm" by ECG) is given as 60 to 100 bpm. However, sustained resting rates above 90 per minute in adults are actually fast and may be a clue to an important diagnosis, such as pulmonary embolism, heart failure, hyperthyroidism, infection, drug effects, anxiety, pain, or hypovolemia leading to shock. [Failure of the pulse to slow and blood pressure to "dip" during periods of non-REM (rapid eye movement) sleeping time is also abnormal. However, chronobiologic dynamics are rarely cited clinically.]

UNDER PRESSURE

Like heart rate, system arterial blood pressure (BP) is a dynamic variable. This is evident when watching the monitor of a patient in the ICU who has a cannulized artery ("art line," usually in a radial artery), and seeing the pressure variation from beat to beat. These values will be recorded in the chart (often called the flow sheet, with other parameters recorded), and the change in these values is often of paramount importance. For example, when a patient with urosepsis is admitted to the intensive care unit because of hypotension, knowing his blood pressure precisely on admission (e.g., 75/40 mmHg) and seeing the response to vasopressors is critical information. When reporting these vital signs, one might describe the BP as a range over time:

> *On admission, the blood pressure range was 65–71/35–47 mmHg, and after being placed on 5 µg/min of intravenous norepinephrine at midnight, it improved to 80–110/50–70. The most recently recorded systemic arterial BP, one hour ago, was 96/60 mmHg.*

By contrast, on the wards, blood pressure (although still constantly in flux) is recorded—with a manual or automated BP cuff—only at a specified interval (e.g., every 8 hours, or every shift change). For example, one might report:

The blood pressure in the emergency department at 7:00 p.m. was 100/60 mmHg. The blood pressure when he arrived on the floor at 8:00 p.m. after receiving a bolus of 1 L of normal saline had improved to 125/75 mmHg. Overnight, the range was 113–143/64–81 mmHg.

Finally, it is always recommended to repeat the blood pressure reading yourself with a manual cuff, especially if the values seem amiss. In addition, vital signs are dynamic—you may find that a patient may not be hypertensive and tachycardic when you repeat the vitals, which were taken initially after the patient rushed to an out-patient clinic visit from the parking lot, half a mile away. Repeating the initial BP and heart rate often yields values closer to "baseline." Vital signs in the emergency department may change strikingly after admission and even during the initial evaluation process. For outpatient follow-up, serial BP measurements, if accurate, can be invaluable to check for "white coat" effects and to avoid overmedication. The accuracy of these measurements can be validated by having the patient bring his or her monitor to the office and simultaneously checking the two measurements. (How do you validate the accuracy of the sphygmomanometers that you rely on?)

FINDING HIDDEN INFORMATION IN VITAL SIGNS— MORE ADVANCED ANALYSIS

The description above presents a kind of "first-order" description of the vital signs. Sometimes, these most fundamental of measurements, which seem very straightforward, contain hidden information that can be extracted by more probing analysis. A few examples are given below.

Pulsus Alternans in Heart Failure

A subtle but important finding in heart failure, usually severe, is alternation of the amplitude of the systolic/diastolic blood pressures on a beat-to-beat basis (ABABAB . . .), usually accompanied by sinus

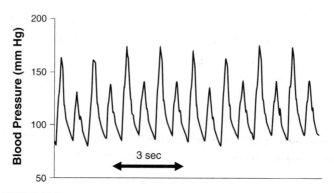

FIGURE 2.3   Pulsus alternans in a patient with heart failure.

tachycardia. This phenomenon, perhaps alluded to in the opening quote by novelist D.H. Lawrence, is called pulsus alternans (Figure 2.3). It has been related to abnormal calcium handling by dysfunctional myocardial cells, but the precise mechanism remains unknown. This finding is difficult to detect by a manual exam, although the savvy examiner may be able to detect alternating changes in the pulse amplitude at the bedside. If your patient is in the ICU or coronary care unit (CCU) with an intraarterial line, you may be able to see alternans on the monitor and record it. But you will notice pulsus alternans only by looking for it. What are the estimated sensitivity and specificity of this sign for the diagnosis of heart failure? The answer is that there is no glib answer. The answers will depend importantly on the severity of the heart failure syndrome and how it is measured (by exam or arterial line). The sign appears to be highly specific but not very sensitive, and its sensitivity goes up as the degree of heart failure worsens. Perhaps you can design a study in the CCU to investigate this question further in patients with arterial lines. While on the subject of pulsus alternans (and connecting with learning techniques in Chapter 11), do you know the meaning and mechanisms of signs with similar names but very different implications, including pulsus paradoxus, electrical alternans, and pulse deficit?

Beyond its association with heart failure, pulsus alternans is important because it exemplifies two general principles of the physical exam:

Principle 1. The physical exam requires an active process of interrogation and hypothesis testing.

Principle 2. The physical exam can be viewed as a series of lab tests. Hence, every physical finding that you seek and either "find" or "do not find" should always prompt you to know or research the estimated sensitivity, specificity, and predictive values of that sign.

Breath-Taking Mistakes

Respiration is probably the single least accurately recorded of the vital signs on the wards and in the clinics. Indeed, in most patients it is unlikely that it is even measured. The patient is quickly inspected and a default "normative" value of 12 to 20 breaths/min is recorded, or perhaps more than 20 if they look more tachypneic. If you want to generate some controversy and discussion, poll your colleagues, students, senior M.D.'s, and nurses on what they consider the normal resting breathing rate.

What is your resting breathing rate? How do you measure it, and does the act of observing yourself change it? Have a colleague measure your breathing rate simultaneously and see if it agrees with your self-measurement. A rate of 20 per minute is sometimes reported, as a kind of default setting, to indicate a normal respiratory rate. Actually, this tempo at rest usually represents tachypnea.

A few comments about commonly confused nomenclature: *Dyspnea* is the subjective sensation of being short of breath, or having difficulty breathing. This term applies to a symptom, not a sign. *Tachypnea*, or rapid breathing rate, is a sign that may be present with or without dyspnea. Thus, a patient may have an abnormally rapid breathing rate at rest and not complain of dyspnea. Conversely, a patient with a respiratory rate in the normal range may complain of considerable shortness of breath. Attendings should be aware of this common misperception and try to correct the terminology when noted.

In order of least acceptable to better, here is how breathing should not be counted:

1. Copy the value on someone else's intake exam. As stated above, in the presence of other "normal" vital signs, a respiratory rate of 20 per minute would be incongruous, or alert the listener to an additional problem or concern that may not be the focus of the chief complaint.
2. Take a look and make a quick estimate.
3. Watch the patient's chest or abdomen for 10 seconds and multiply by 6 to get the rate per minute.

The first two mistakes do not merit further comment. The third seems reasonable. However, watching a patient with your wristwatch or looking at the clock on the wall is awkward and may make you or the patient self-conscious. Further, depending on the degree of abdominal or chest breathing, it may be difficult to tell what is actually a breath, and then you have to start a recount. Also, respiration has a more voluntary component than the other vital signs: we may change the pattern of breathing or rate, or even hold our breath, when we feel we are being observed.

A useful clinical trick is to combine the respiratory rate calculation with the examination of the neck. Begin by politely ask the patient not to talk. *After auscultating over the carotids and the thyroid for bruits, simply listen over the trachea. Inspiration and expiration cycles are usually quite clear. If you listen for 20 seconds and multiply by 3, a reasonably good average breathing rate is obtained.* (Some clinicians favor counting respirations as unobtrusively as possible in concert with measuring the pulse rate.)

Another source of error is to miss central (*Cheyne–Stokes breathing*) or obstructive sleep apnea at the bedside (Figure 2.4). The reason is that with these common breathing abnormalities the rate changes dramatically over 30 seconds to 1 minute from relatively fast to zero if there is a frank apnea. Most clinical observers are understandably loath to record the breathing rate as zero, so if they are measuring respiration with periodic breathing they will wait until the patient has started breathing again, which will lead to an overestimate of the breathing rate. (One clue to this is seeing a recorded rate of 30 to 40 in a patient who is not in respiratory distress.) In a patient

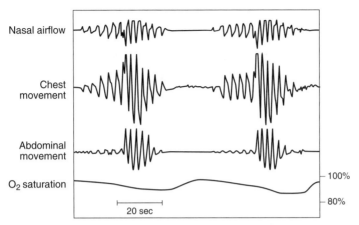

FIGURE 2.4 Periodic (Cheyne–Stokes) breathing. What is the respiratory rate? The answer is that the conventional notation of the number of breaths per minute is not meaningful here. Instead are the patient's breathing cycles between slower and shallower breaths, culminating in an apneic period, and then faster and deeper breaths. This condition is most common in heart failure but may also be seen in other settings, including stroke and aging. A distinct but similar pattern of variable breathing occurs with obstructive sleep apnea.

with periodic breathing, you should not record an average rate but, instead, note that respirations reveal periodic breathing, and, if you can, give a time to the duration of the apparent apneic phases (e.g., 15 seconds).

As you get more sophisticated, you will be able to detect pure obstructive apneas—with increased respiratory effort but no airflow—from pure central apneas where respiratory effort ceases periodically. However, keep in mind that many patients have mixed (complex) apneas that combine both mechanisms. *Simply recognizing period-type breathing at the bedside will make you appear to be an Oslerian wizard.* Be on the lookout for Cheyne–Stokes breathing in a patient with severe heart failure.

Always treat the physical exam as an active process. Experienced clinicians look and listen *for*, not *at* or *to*.

For intubated patients in intensive care units, mention should be made of the mode of ventilation, the respiratory rate (displayed on the ventilator), whether the patient is "overbreathing" the rate set by the ventilator, and other programmable features (e.g., positive end-expiratory pressure). Students should make more use of this visual display of data, which can help make their exams more objective and help take advantage of information not readily obtained by the traditional physical exam.

Comparison with Previous Values

Any clinically important difference between a current vital sign and a baseline value, if available, must be flagged and noted in your presentation and write-up; for example, *Mr. Paulsen's weight is 83 kg compared with 72 kg reported three weeks ago.* This statement motivates key follow-up questions: Is the increase real, in which case almost certainly due to marked fluid accumulation? Or, is it spurious, due to one or both values being erroneous, or inconsistent due to clothing?

REPLACING SEMI- OR PSEUDOQUANTITATIVE MEASURES WITH MORE USEFUL QUALITATIVE MEASURES

Science is said to aspire to be more quantitative, not less. However, the connection of science with strict quantification is valid only if the measures have some meaningful, consistent, and reproducible interpretation. For many clinical aspects of the physical exam, we have come to use relatively meaningless or at best confusing semiquantitative measures.

A good example is answering the question: *How much pedal edema does my patient have?* Pedal edema is an important finding in multiple pathological conditions, including heart failure, renal failure, hepatic failure, primary venous insufficiency, and venous or lymphatic disease due to thrombosis or tumor. However, some degree of pedal edema can be a false positive due to physiological or clinically inconsequential venous insufficiency (e.g., mild lower extremity swelling after a prolonged period of standing).

The common practice of scoring edema on a scale of 0 to 5+ is essentially meaningless if there is no consensus on what this index means to you compared to your colleagues. What if your 5+ and my 4+ are identical and our 1+ scores are different? How do you circumvent the problem of scoring the amount of pedal edema in a simple, reproducible, yet meaningful way, a subject that is almost never taught in physical diagnosis courses? A useful solution to this problem is to qualitatively rate pedal edema as *trace*, *mild*, *moderate*, and *marked*, and then actually measure an area at a given level relative to the ankles and record the circumference of this pedal region in centimeters. In this way, the next observer who comes to the bedside can replicate your measurements, + or − the inherent error in the measure. You can accommodate this standard error by approximating and writing "~cm." Perhaps you can think of an alternative way to add rigor to this everyday measurement. You can start by doing a simple study of observer variability in rating of pedal edema on the wards.

How Should You Grade a Cardiac Murmur?

Clinicians too often toss around phrases like "I heard a grade II systolic/diastolic murmur" without any additional information. Such a statement is not very helpful or informative. What can you say that will be meaningful? You should give not only the intensity of murmurs but also state the patient's position (supine, left lateral decubitus, sitting, squatting, etc.), the quality (soft, harsh, blowing, etc.), and the specified anatomical location (e.g., left parasternal area or apex); a change with position (e.g., aortic insufficiency murmurs are often heard best and louder when the patient leans forward, and a murmur of hypertrophic obstructive cardiomyopathy may increase with a Valsalva maneuver); and finally, the temporal nature of the murmur (early, mid, or late systolic, holosystolic, diastolic, etc.). Savvy listeners may comment on the "dynamics" of the murmur, such as crescendo–decrescendo, or late-peaking.

In this instance, it is perfectly appropriate, and perhaps even preferable, to rate the intensity of the murmur in one of three categories: soft, moderate, or loud. A reasonable statement would be:

> *I heard a moderately loud, blowing holosystolic (pansystolic) murmur most evident in the anterior axillary area with the patient in the left lateral decubitus position.*

A cardiologist listening to this report would be grateful for a rigorous description of a probable mitral regurgitant murmur. However, she or he will keep in mind the possibility that it could also be the description of an aortic stenosis murmur with the high-frequency components being transmitted preferentially to the apex, a finding referred to as the *Gallavardin phenomenon.*

> The murmur of aortic stenosis may change in quality and become musical in its propagation to the cardiac apex.
> —JEAN PIERRE GALLAVARDIN (1875–1957)

The Gallavardin sign is interesting from a more general physical diagnosis point of view in that it illustrates a phenomenon that simultaneously reduces the sensitivity of the exam for one diagnosis (possibly missing aortic stenosis) and decreasing the specificity for another (false-positive sign of mitral regurgitation).

Another example of a useful statement could be:

> *I heard a soft blowing diastolic murmur in the right parasternal area that was best appreciated with the patient holding her breath and leaning forward.*

This finding would be classic for aortic regurgitation.

Use of the official American Heart Association grading system of 1–6/6 is useful only if you know what the numbers actually mean. Since most observers in training do not, calling a murmur 4/6 when it is actually 2/6 is misleading. Of note, young or less experienced examiners may not hear or barely hear a murmur and thereby undercall it, while that same murmur will be clearly audible to a more experienced auscultator.

Caution for Attendings: Eponyms and Acronyms—Avoiding Useless Physical Finding Archaic Digressions during Rounds Every practitioner would like to have some finding named for herself or himself. Eponynmous designations— Ewart's sign, Beck's triad, Murphy's sign, Gallavardin's sign—convey a type of clinical immortality (assuming, of course, that you know who the person being referenced is). And indeed, for actual diseases—Alzheimer's disease, Lesch–Nyhan syndrome, Creutzfeldt–Jakob disease, to name but a few—the discoverers and the disease states have become eponymously synonymous.

Where attending rounds get bogged down is in asking about outmoded acronyms that have little or no contemporary relevance. Some of the best examples are terms dating back a century or more for findings of severe aortic regurgitation (insufficiency): Corrigan's water hammer pulse, de Musset's head nodding, Traube's pistol shot, Duroziez's sign, and so on. These signs are all related to widened pulse pressure and increased stroke volume, key features of the pathophysiology of very severe, chronic aortic valve regurgita-tion, dating back to the era when untreated syphilitic aortitis and rheumatic disease were leading cardiac diagnoses.

However, for the most part, these terms have become historical relics. They have little or no relevance to modern practice, in which most aortic insufficiency is much more subtle and may be evidenced only by an easily overlooked diastolic blowing murmur (heard with the patient holding his breath and leaning forward or squatting), which sounds more like a whisper than a true auscultatory event. By the time someone has head nodding or femoral pistol shots, the patient usually has nearly wide-open chronic insufficiency with a very loud diastolic murmur and a wide pulse pressure.

Quizzing students and house staff about ancient eponymous signs is one of the reasons that the physical exam has mistakenly been thought to have become outmoded.

For those who are interested, the official rating system of heart murmurs appears in Table 2.1. Important to note, but not well appre-ciated, is the fact that the same grading system is used for systolic, diastolic, and continuous murmurs. However, it is becoming increas-ingly common to grade diastolic murmurs based on a 4-point scale, given that they are rarely above 3/6 in intensity.

Caution: If someone says that he or she is hearing a 4/4–6 diastolic murmur, there is a good chance that this statement is in error—

TABLE 2.1   Gradations of Cardiac Murmurs

Grade	Description
1	Very faint, heard only after listener has "tuned in"; may not be heard in all positions
2	Quiet, but heard immediately after placing the stethoscope on the chest
3	Moderately loud
4	Loud, with palpable thrill (i.e., a tremor or buzzy vibration felt on palpation)
5	Very loud, with thrill; may be heard when stethoscope is partly off the chest
6	Very loud, with thrill; may be heard with stethoscope entirely off the chest

Source: American Heart Association.

perhaps it is a systolic murmur, perhaps it is an artifact, or perhaps it is a loud diastolic murmur that is overrated as to intensity.

What Is the CVP? How Would You RSVP?

Central venous pressure (CVP) (Figure 2.5) is yet another example where pseudoquantitation is more the rule than the exception. CVP is a key indicator of cardiopulmonary physiology and pathophysiology as well as of overall volume status. Attempts to measure CVP *at the bedside of the mean CVP are perhaps the least reliable numbers generated in a routine exam.* Indeed, when applied to CVP, the term *measures* is a misnomer, as these numbers are at best estimates. "Evidence-based" studies of CVP, nicely summarized by Dr. Deborah J. Cook and Dr. David J. Simel in their 1996 *JAMA* article, confirmed poor sensitivities and specificities for this vital part of the exam when compared with actual hemodynamic measurements.

   At least five factors are responsible for this confusion and for substantial errors that may affect patient management:

   1. Probably very few students or house officers know what the relevant units are for this measure. The CVP as measured at

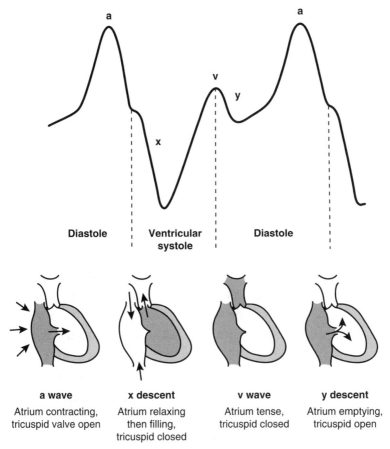

FIGURE 2.5 Sequential phases of central venous pressure. Two major positive waves (a and v) are present with two negative deflections (x and y) related to atrial and ventricular hemodynamics. These waves and descents are very challenging, even for experts, to decipher at the bedside. They are best analyzed as printouts (requiring an indwelling catheter in the right atrium), with a concomitant ECG recording. From Longmore M, Wilkinson I, Torok E (eds.). The Oxford Handbook of Clinical Medicine, 5th Ed. Oxford, UK: Oxford University Press, 2001, p. 79. Reproduced with permission.

the bedside by exam is in millimeters or centimeters of blood. The CVP recorded from ICU monitors is likely recorded in mmHg, or sometimes in cm H_2O (if a saline-filled manometer is used). The conversion factor between the two is 1 mmHg = 1.36 cm H_2O.

2. Although the external jugular veins are used routinely (which some clinicians feel is acceptable), the CVP ideally should be estimated from the *right internal* jugular veins and estimated in various positions to assure accuracy. If the external jugular vein is the only one you can visualize, this fact should be noted in the presentation.

3. The CVP should be obtained relative to the center of the right atrium, which is not possible to locate reliably at the bedside. As noted by Dr. Jules Constant in his classic book, *Bedside Cardiology*, the CVP is usually measured relative to the sternal angle with the head of the patient's bed inclined at 45°. The upper normal limit for the CVP at this angle is about 4.5 cm of blood. "Some cardiologists insist on adding an assumed distance of 5 cm between the bottom of the right atrium and the sternal angle to make the upper normal 9.5 cm of blood. This seems to be an unnecessary additional step, since the distance between the right atrium and the sternal angle is really an unknown factor."

4. The absolute value of the CVP is only one of four relevant parameters of central venous hemodynamics, which also include (a) the response to respiration, (b) the morphology of the pulse curves, and (c) abdominojugular reflux (previously and sometimes still termed hepatojugular reflux), the response to gentle but firm midabdominal pressure.*

5. Perhaps most important, very high pressures due to severe heart failure are often missed because the meniscus (top) of the fluid wave may be above the jaw, even with the patient

---

*Failure of the CVP to fall upon inspiration is an indicator of reduced right heart compliance and is seen in three major contexts of severe diastolic dysfunction: restrictive cardiomyopathies such as cardiac amyloidosis or sarcoidosis, constrictive pericarditis, and right ventricular infarction. The morphology of the waves (A, V, and the X and Y descents) is complex and very difficult to assess at the bedside, even for experts, without a waveform recording. Sustained elevation of the CVP with upper abdominal pressure, and failure to fall after pressure is released, are markers of reduced right heart compliance.

sitting upright, so that a falsely low value is recorded. This oversight is a serious error since marked elevation of the CVP indicates a life-threatening problem (Figure 2.5). On the other hand, mistaking the carotid pulse for the jugular pulse can lead to false-positive estimates of elevated central venous pressure.

Finally, it should be mentioned that the neck vein examination is extremely challenging, even to seasoned practitioners. In your early stages of training, simply being able to assess whether the CVP is normal, high, or low is an accomplishment.

Key Parameters of Central Venous Pressure

1. *Amplitude.* Is it low, normal, or elevated, and if so, how elevated? The key question is whether the pressure is low, normal, or high.
2. *Response to respiration.* Of use primarily when the pressure appears elevated.
3. *Waveform morphology.* A and V waves and X and Y descents (Figure 2.5). For most observers, the only waveform abnormality that is likely to be noted is a prominent V wave—indicating tricuspid regurgitation. Other findings usually require actual CVP tracing.
4. *Abdominojugular reflux.* Variability is introduced by nonstandard degrees and durations of abdominal pressure and by interpretation of neck findings.

EXAMPLE

A 51-year-old man had recurrent presentations to the urgent care clinic because of increasing lower extremity edema and abdominal girth. He reported that this swelling began five years ago. He denied consuming alcohol for over 10 years but carried the diagnosis of hepatic cirrhosis due to alcohol. He was usually discharged with diuretics, which were only modestly helpful in relieving his symptoms. On one of his presentations, a newly minted intern performed a physical examination and was the first observer to report marked jugular venous distention, a finding *not* consistent with alcoholic cirrhosis. Further history taking revealed that he was admitted to an outside hospital with pericarditis six years earlier.

Intracardiac pressure measurements obtained during cardiac catheterization revealed a mean right atrial pressure of 15 mmHg, right ventricular pressure of 65/16 mmHg, left ventricular pressure of 145/16 mmHg, and mean pulmonary capillary wedge pressure of 16 mmHg (indicating elevation and near equalization of diastolic filling pressures), along with a classic "dip and plateau pattern in the right ventricular pressure trace," also known as the "square root sign" (Figure 2.6). These findings were strongly suggestive of constrictive pericarditis, most often caused by severe calcification of the pericardium, probably secondary to his prior pericarditis. Cardiac magnetic resonance imaging showed pericardial calcification along the visceral and parietal pericardium. The patient underwent surgical pericardiectomy with resolution of his symptoms.

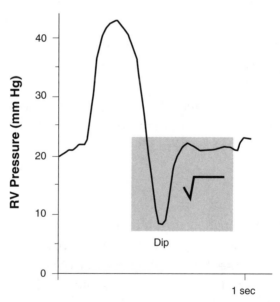

FIGURE 2.6 Right ventricular pressure tracing in constrictive pericarditis with the square root sign.

Comment: The correct and lifesaving diagnosis here was reached only by readdressing a history that had been propagated via chart lore and possibly cut-and-paste write-ups. The re-look was prompted by a physical exam by an unbiased new team member that revealed an outlier finding (Chapter 10): prominent jugular venous distention. The often-subtle but critical finding subverted the long-held diagnosis of alcoholic cirrhosis (or would have required two diseases, e.g., cardiomyopathy and cirrhosis) and led, finally, to the correct diagnosis of constrictive pericarditis.

INCREASING YOUR LEVEL OF CERTAINTY: INTERNAL CONFIRMATIONS

When you make an assessment on exam, such as CVP amplitude or hepatic enlargement, how confident can you be that the finding or the estimate of its magnitude is reasonably valid? You can employ at least three complementary approaches to increase your level of certainty:

1. Intraobserver checking (self-replication)
2. Multimodal testing
3. Interobserver checking

The easiest way to increase your level of certainty is simply to go back to see if the findings are reproducible. Reproducibility is a central aspect of the scientific method. The physical exam is a series of complex, interwoven mini-tests and hypothesis-testing exercises. Can you replicate your own findings? In the case of measurements such as CVP, checking them in different positions is very helpful. The meniscus of visible venous waves should decrease as the patient sits more upright. A second strategy, when available, is to use relatively independent (multimodal) techniques to confirm a finding. A good example is in the estimation of hepatic size. There are at least three methods: percussion, palpation, and the "scratch test." It is very reassuring if the estimated boundaries of the liver are comparable using all three. A third approach is to ask for a second opinion from a colleague blinded to your call.

Keep in mind, however, that some findings are notoriously unstable and evanescent, such as pericardial friction rubs, which may come and go and are often position dependent. Not hearing a rub at one time and hearing it later, or vice versa, does not disprove its existence. Having an independent observer confirm a finding that may be transient is very helpful.

When feasible, use imaging to test your hypotheses developed on physical exam—for example, heart size with chest x-ray and echocardiogram, murmurs with the latter; thyroid size and nodularity with appropriate scans; liver, abdominal aortic aneurysm, and liver/spleen sizes with ultrasound or other modalities. The teaching benefit of these tests for refining physical diagnostic skills is vastly underutilized and deserves more rigorous studies.

PHYSICAL EXAM: SEMANTIC AND SCIENTIFIC PRECISION

One of the themes of this book on the *interstitial curriculum* is the paucity of attention paid to addressing uncertainty in all aspects of medicine, well beyond the notions of sensitivity, specificity, and predictive values of a given physical finding or lab test. On the one hand, we would like to purge uncertainty from our judgments to make them as scientific and error-proof as possible. Yet, as we have seen, the science itself is based, from the micro to the macro levels, on varied sources of uncertainty. In some respects, medicine is definable as the science of uncertainty as applied to health and disease.

The collision of fact with physical finding can be unsettling, as, for example, when you state that there was no "organomegaly," but the abdominal ultrasound reveals hepatosplenomegaly. Students should be led away from making statements such as "no murmurs were heard" or "the thyroid was normal" to making more scientifically accurate ones, such as "I did not hear any murmurs" and "To my exam, the thyroid was not enlarged and without nodules." Similarly, a more rigorous statement is always that "no organomegaly was appreciated or detected by palpation." Such statements accommodate the limitations of the particular examiner and of the physical examination in general.

Attending's Perspective: The Physical Exam

The performance and presentation of the physical exam by students and house staff pose major challenges for attendings. These are analogous to those discussed at the end of Chapter 1 regarding the history. A major preoccupation is assessing the validity and reliability of the findings and deciding which ones need the most careful rechecking and vetting. It is important to encourage the students' and residents' examination skills and commitment to their findings, as it is increasingly common to place more emphasis and complete reliance on noninvasive imaging studies (e.g., CT scans, transthoracic echocardiograms), with the pernicious side effect of deemphasizing the importance of the exam. Bedside rounds can be an excellent opportunity for reevaluation with concomitant evidence-based teaching.

MINI-SUMMARY

- Every exam must begin with a general assessment of the patient.
- All physical signs have sensitivities and specificities—indeed, they are lab test equivalents.
- The vital signs are often measured incompletely and recorded inaccurately.
- You can count the respiration rate accurately by auscultating over the trachea for 30 seconds or 1 minute and in this way can also make a diagnosis of Cheyne–Stokes (periodic) breathing.
- The physical exam is an active iterative process. Try to focus your exam on the clinical context of the patient being examined. Look, feel, and listen *for*, not *to*.
- Consider the exam to be a series of hypothesis-testing exercises.
- Try to confirm physical findings using an independent method (e.g., percussion, palpation, the scratch test for assessing liver

span); also, see if you can replicate your findings and whether colleagues, blinded to your assessment, observe the same or different findings.

- Avoid statements such as *No organomegaly was present on abdominal exam* in favor of more scientific observations such as *I did not feel an enlarged spleen or liver with palpation of the abdomen.*

CHAPTER 3

HOW (NOT) TO ORDER
AND PRESENT LAB TESTS

Confusion now hath made his masterpiece.
                    —WILLIAM SHAKESPEARE (1564–1616), from *Macbeth*

Note to Attendings and Residents: The following discussion gives our preferences in lab test reporting. We recommend that upon assuming management of a ward service, you give your team guidance as to how you prefer tests and related findings to be presented.

After presenting of the history and physical, your next focus should be a summary of key admission and follow-up laboratory tests. Sometimes one or more of these tests has been mentioned in the history as part of the reason that the patient was admitted (e.g., right lower lung field density on chest x-ray, positive blood cultures). However, a small amount of (appropriate) repetition is not only acceptable but desirable in most clinical presentations.

The tests that are ordered as part of the initial assessment depend largely on the specific reason for admission, but usually include certain "routine" tests as well. The latter are justified for providing baseline information or because they may reveal a hidden abnormality that could be relevant to future management. More often than

---

Becoming a Consummate Clinician: What Every Student, House Officer, and Hospital Practitioner Needs to Know, First Edition.
Ary L. Goldberger and Zachary D. Goldberger.
© 2012 Wiley-Blackwell. Published 2012 by John Wiley & Sons, Inc.

not, a set of routine or baseline labs are ordered a priori once a patient is admitted or is seen in the emergency department. *However, as a rule, no tests should be considered routine. Additional laboratory testing or imaging studies may add cost and the possibility of detecting false-positive results that may engender needless and sometimes dangerous follow-up testing or examinations.* Attendings should encourage and even instigate debates about such questions as "Why did we order this test?" and "What were the alternatives?"

As a general rule, adopt a "zero-based" attitude toward ordering lab tests: Be able to explain why each test is relevant, what you would do with a positive result, and the alternatives.

EXAMPLE

You are the admitting resident on call and also, unfortunately, scheduled to be in your outpatient continuity clinic that afternoon. Your last appointment is with Steven Smith, a 37-year-old new patient who has recently moved to the area and wishes to establish medical care. He has no complaints, and his past medical history is remarkable only for a tonsillectomy as a child and seasonal allergic rhinitis, for which he takes over-the-counter loratidine as needed. His family history is remarkable for a paternal grandfather who had a myocardial infarction in his 70s; both his parents are alive and well. He has never smoked, drinks two or three glasses of wine per week, and is married with three young children. He works as an engineer for a major car manufacturer. He exercises vigorously three times a week without difficulty. His vaccinations are up to date.

On examination, he is friendly and well-appearing. Vital signs are normal. The remainder of his examination is unremarkable. You decide that he should have one set of "routine" labs, including a serum chemistry panel ("Chem-7") and a complete blood count.

You return to the hospital to begin admitting new inpatients. At 10:00 p.m., the outpatient laboratory pages you and informs you that Mr. Smith has serum sodium of 115 mEq/L. The reason for this, you suspect, is lab error. Mr. Smith had no symptoms of hyponatremia (altered mental status, muscle weakness, nausea, headache) and an extremely low prior probability of any condition associated with this finding (e.g., syndrome of inappropriate antidiuretic hormone). However, since this finding constitutes an abnormal and "critical" lab value, you call Mr. Smith and explain that he needs to return to the emergency department for a repeat lab draw. The repeat check was 138 mEq/L.

This case illustrates the point that no lab tests should be considered routine, even if ordered routinely in specific contexts, such as preop testing or upon general hospital admission. The central message is that even though he was a new outpatient without recorded labs, many clinicians (supported by the U.S. Preventive Services Task Force Recommendations) would vigorously argue that a 37-year-old man with an unremarkable history and a normal physical examination has no hard indication for general screening laboratory tests, with the exception of a fasting lipid panel. For inpatients, guidelines regarding routine test ordering are not practicable given the huge range of conditions leading to such hospital admissions.

"INCIDENTAL" FINDINGS

Finally, there is the issue of "incidentalomas," apparent "findings" usually on imaging studies that appear abnormal, yet were not related to why you ordered the study (see also Chapter 12).

EXAMPLE

A 56-year-old man with a 50-pack-year history of smoking and mild COPD is admitted to your service for shortness of breath, thought to be an exacerbation of his COPD. The chest x-ray performed in the ED did not show any focal infiltrates suspicious for pneumonia or other acute process. Exam reveals rhonchi and expiratory wheezes. You order one treatment of nebulized albuterol and one dose of 60 mg IV solumedrol. Initially he feels better, with less dyspnea. Overnight, however, he complains of sharp left-sided pleuritic chest pain. No rub is heard on exam. An ECG reveals no signs of acute ischemia or pericarditis. Cardiac troponins are negative. You send the patient for a high-resolution chest CT with contrast to evaluate for pulmonary embolism (PE). An hour later, you receive a call from the radiologist, who says that the study is negative for PE but reveals a 3- to 4-mm, noncalcified nodule in the left lower lobe.

How would you manage this finding? As a fortuitous discovery or as an incidental distraction? Given the patient's risk factors for lung cancer, he may be subject to follow-up CT scans, with the risks of repeat radiation for what may turn out to be a nonfinding. But perhaps one test that was negative for the primary concern uncovered a new finding that itself might lead to lifesaving intervention. Incidental findings of this kind are becoming more frequent with the enhanced quality of medical imaging.

Note to Attendings. A useful exercise during rounds is to go through mini-drills in which you ask team members two key questions:

1. What are you looking for from a given test?
2. What will you do if the test shows a given finding? For example, "You said you ordered a set of 'lytes.' What will you do if the serum sodium returns at 120 mEq/L?"

Clinicians should always expect the unexpected when ordering lab tests. The following general principles are suggested as guides to ordering and following up on lab tests.

Four C's of Lab Test Ordering: Contribution; Contingency; Compliance; Communication

1. Only order tests that *contribute* to diagnosis, prognosis, or management. A shotgun approach may leave both you and your patient with shrapnel. For example, if you are thinking of

ordering a bone densitometry study on a middle-aged female patient, but no change in management will be enacted regardless of the findings, don't order it.

2. Always formulate a *contingency* game plan ("what if . . .") based on what the test might show. "What will I do if the acid phosphatase is mildly elevated? Markedly elevated? Upper limits of normal?"

3. Develop a "flagging" mechanism to ensure that tests ordered are actually performed, or find out how these tests are followed in your own practice. Just because you order a test, especially in an outpatient setting, doesn't mean that the patient will actually *comply* and have that test.

4. Always have a plan for *communicating* the results of the test both to the patient and other caregivers as appropriate. Failure to follow up on biopsy or lab tests is unacceptable medicine and has major medicolegal consequences.

A complete blood count (CBC) is obtained universally in *major* medical and surgical admissions. An electrocardiogram (ECG or EKG; Figure 3.1), in contrast, is generally reserved for patients with a history or complaint relevant to the cardiovascular system, or in those who, because of advanced age or the presence of other disease processes, are at risk of important abnormalities that may otherwise be unrecognized (e.g., prior "silent" myocardial infarction). In other

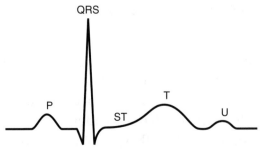

FIGURE 3.1 Basic ECG waveforms (lead II).

cases, an ECG on hospital admission may serve as a comparative baseline for cardiac complications of subsequent therapy (e.g., prior to potentially cardiotoxic chemotherapy).

The major justification for obtaining routine ECGs in asymptomatic patients is to detect an unrecognized or "silent" myocardial infarction (Figure 3.1). The incidence of this possibility goes up with age and with certain comorbidities, such as diabetes mellitus and possibly hypertension. Thus, an admission ECG would usually be considered part of routine assessment in a 75-year-old man admitted with lower abdominal pain but not in an otherwise healthy 30-year-old woman with acute pyelonephritis and normal renal function.

Furthermore, some laboratory testing may actually be cost-saving, due largely to prevention of unnecessary hospital admission. For example, B-type natriuretic peptide (BNP), a protein released by the left ventricle in response to stretch, may be helpful in distinguishing between dyspnea due to decompensated heart failure versus another less severe process (e.g., exacerbation of chronic obstructive pulmonary disease). Early investigations with BNP suggested a decrease in hospital admissions, the median length of stay, and average total cost of treatment (Mueller C, et al. N Engl J Med. 2004;350:647–654) due to the discovery of an alternative diagnosis for shortness of breath not requiring aggressive inpatient management. However, a normal BNP does not exclude other life-threatening causes of dyspnea, including acute pulmonary embolism. Laboratory tests must always be interpreted in the full clinical context, with appreciation of their diagnostic uses and limitations.

CLASSIFICATION OF BASIC LAB DATA

Exhibit 3.1 presents a simple classification of the lab data you order routinely. The data fall into two major groups: (1) noninvasive or minimally invasive, and (2) invasive. Within each group are subdivisions. When presenting the labs, it is good practice to present tests beginning with the least invasive and ending with the more invasive, generally in the order in which they are obtained and of their clinical

EXHIBIT 3.1 How to Classify Basic Laboratory Tests: Examples

A. Noninvasive or minimally invasive
   Body fluid analysis: blood, sputum, urine
   Imaging studies: standard x-rays, ultrasound data (including echocardiograms and abdominal ultrasounds), computerized tomographic data, magnetic resonance data, positron emission tomographic data
   Electrocardiogram and other cardiac signal data: Holter monitors, event recorders (including both automatic and patient-activated)
   Neurophysiologic signal data: electroencephalogram, polysomnogram, electromyogram
B. Invasive
   Cavity fluid "centeses": pleural, ascitic, joint, pericardial, cerebrospinal
   Cardiac catheterization; coronary angiography
   Peripheral vessel and cerebral angiography
   Aspirates and biopsies (e.g., bone marrow, breast; other needle biopsies)
   Bronchoscopy-related studies
   Endoscopy/colonoscopy-related studies

priority in a given case. For example, a reasonable way to proceed in a patient with clinical evidence of a new cerebrovascular event would be presenting the CBC, prothrombin time or partial thromboplastin time, relevant chemistries, and ECG followed by the detailed neuro-imaging evaluation. Skipping over the CBC, say, for the sake of efficiency, might lead to ignoring evidence of polycythemia vera or thrombocytosis, which might be of etiological importance; thrombocytopenia or anemia might affect the decision to initiate anticoagulant or thrombolytic therapy for a thromboembolic stroke.

PRESENTATION OF LAB TESTS: THE TWO MAJOR PROBLEMS

Two major sources of confusion and error afflict the presentation of lab tests:

1. Inconsistent and illogical presentation of the findings, here termed the "zigzag" presentation
2. Incomplete sourcing and validation of primary data

Zigzag Labs

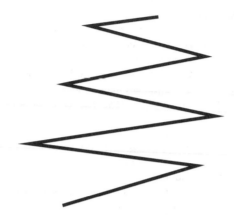

Zigzagging: not the way to present lab data.

While *zigzagging* is a good way to deliberately lose someone whom you do *not* want to follow you—a proven strategy to throw someone off the trail—it is exactly the opposite in clinical presentations, where efficient flow of information is of paramount importance. One major and avoidable problem in your presentation of the lab exam is the failure to provide a consistent framework on which to display these key data. A common student and house staff pitfall is to recite the labs in a nearly random order (and in one that changes from one presentation to the next). While Ralph Waldo Emerson in his essay "Self-Reliance" pronounced a "foolish consistency" to be the "hobgoblin of little minds," the lack of a flexible but consistent organization impairs communication. You should have a relatively standard way of organizing and presenting lab data, and attendings should insist on this type of presentational "infrastructure."

Experienced clinicians are accustomed to hearing about lab tests in a fairly stylized way. This "anticipatory posture" promotes attention and allows for critical listening. (You may want to argue that your senior attendings or department chairs are too rigid, but that argument is one you are not likely to win, at least not in the context of how to present data.) The first anticipated component of the lab exam is the CBC, followed by the fundamental blood chemistries. However, if you start your presentation by giving the serum ceruloplasmin, even in a patient for whom Wilson's disease (hepatolenticular degeneration) is a key part of the differential diagnosis, you risk confusing and probably annoying the most important subset of your audience. More important, this type of ad hoc or short-circuited presentation leads to errors in communication and workup that can adversely affect patient care. Of course, in the case of Wilson's disease, hemolytic anemia is an important component, so leaving out the CBC would be a major omission.

Flow of information is a key to efficiency and communication during clinical presentations on rounds and is an important way of reducing errors (Chapter 7). You want your listeners to track you actively, anticipate your next move, and follow your trail of reasoning.

Expedited Presentations

In some settings, an expedited presentation is needed, as opposed to more formal attending rounds and conferences. In these cases it is perfectly acceptable to state that lab tests were "remarkable for the following" and then state the most pertinent positives and negatives. For example: *The CBC was remarkable for a WBC count of 19,000 with 85% neutrophils and 20% lymphocytes, a platelet count of 260,000, and a normal hemoglobin of 14.0 mg/dL—aside from the WBC, these are unchanged from those checked two months ago when he presented after a dog bite. The chemistry panel was remarkable for a BUN of 49 and a creatinine of 1.9. Electrolytes were otherwise normal, and unchanged from labs checked two months ago as well. Urinalysis was negative.* This presentation, although more complete than many you will hear, eliminates some of the other labs that may have been ordered (liver function tests, prothrombin time, calcium) but that are *not* relevant to the particular case being presented.

Outsourcing the Data

A second major source of problems with clinical presentation of lab data is the lack of adequate sourcing. Relying on secondary accounts may be necessary, especially in acute settings, but should always be indicated in the record. The challenges of assessing the validity of test reports are discussed in more depth in Chapter 4. In medicine, as in other scientific settings, seeing (along with data sourced from other senses: hearing, palpating, etc.) is the basis of believing. Accounts by others that you cannot verify should always raise a question mark.

Clinical data presentations are subject to the same flaws that afflict historical and journalistic accounts: namely, identifying the source and verifying the information for labs that weight heavily on diagnosis and management. To give some commonplace examples, consider the following contrasting presentations from three cases.

Case 1: 70-Year-Old Woman with Fever and Cough

Version 1: Chest x-ray on admission was notable for a left lower lung field infiltrate.

Version 2: Chest *PA and lateral* x-ray on admission were notable for the radiologist's reading of a left lower lung field infiltrate. *I reviewed the actual film with the radiologist on call and confirmed this finding with her, with the differential diagnosis of pneumonia, pulmonary infarct, and old fibrosis vs. atelectasis. No previous film was available for comparison. We are calling the primary physician to see if there are any other x-rays from the office or from other institutions available for comparison.*

Case 2: 25-Year-Old Man with Fever and Lymphadenopathy

Version 1: CBC was notable for a total white count of 15,000, with 70% polys and 25% lymphocytes.

Version 2: CBC was reported by the lab as showing an initial white count of 15,000 with 70% polys. *We reviewed the slide with one of the senior technicians and it appears that the automated detector labeled a substantial number of atypical lymphocytes as polys, which suggests the possibility of acute mononucleosis. The count is being redone manually.*

Case 3: 60-Year-Old Man with Chest Discomfort

> *Version 1:* The patient underwent an exercise test that was negative.
>
> *Version 2:* The patient underwent *a stress test that reportedly showed that he performed 14 minutes of treadmill exercise to a heart rate of 150 beats/min, with a normal blood pressure response and with no reported chest discomfort. This is a preliminary report from the person who supervised the exam.*

In each of these examples, the versions with somewhat greater detail place the diagnosis in more direct context and help clarify management plans. A CBC that was overread as mononucleosis would preclude the use of antibiotics. A stress test that was negative for inducible ischemia on exercise echocardiogram in a patient able to exercise to 85% of his maximal heart rate in 14 minutes conveys more prognostic information than data from a patient who was able to exercise for only 3 minutes.

CHECKING PRIMARY SOURCES VS. COPING WITH WORK (OVER) FLOW PRESSURES

The pressure to admit, treat, and discharge patients in a short time period (*high-throughput medicine*) puts a premium on your time and makes it increasingly difficult for students, house officers, and attendings to review primary data. However, the unavoidable competition between increasing reliance on technology (e.g., imaging studies) and the inability to review all of the relevant studies personally is where teamwork is of enormous benefit. For example, deploying medical students to review imaging studies with radiology staff can be of major value, not just in education but in clinical management, and can sometimes lead to reassessment of the findings and to better integration of members of the extended caregiving network. From a student's perspective, the review of primary data with a specialist or consultant can be invaluable and, hopefully, not perceived inappropriately as "scut work."

Attending's Perspective: Freeze-Framing the Lab Test Presentation

In Chapter 3 we introduced freeze-framing, a strategy designed to interrupt a presentation in order to discuss the differential diagnosis or some mechanistic consideration. These moments are sometimes referred to as "getting people out of their comfort zone." However, the intent is not to irritate or play roundsmanship games—quite the opposite. Think of them as teaching enhancements, mechanisms for opening up and enlarging discussions, achieved paradoxically by stopping them temporarily. To avoid the misperception that interruptions are due to poor presentation skills (a separate issue addressed here), you can signal your team at the start of taking service if you are going to employ this style. Also, asking questions to which you yourself don't know the answer fosters the essential notion of teaching rounds as a safe space for scientific questioning and learning.

One important general example is to interrupt presentations about lab test results and ask how a given instrument or testing modality works and what its accuracy is. Trainees and clinicians alike too often take for granted the technology that generates the numbers we use. This *acceptance bias* is especially prevalent in our transmission and recording of routine lab tests (CBCs and chemistry panels are prime examples), the assays that practitioners almost universally assume are valid to the decimal place reported.

In keeping with our previous discussion about the pulse oximeter, sufficient knowledge about the physiology and pathophysiology of medical devices should be required.

> *Attending to student*: "Let's pause for a second. You just said that the fasting glucose was 180 mg/dL. How was that measured?"
>
> *Student*: "By the lab."
>
> *Attending*: "That's where it was measured; but how did the technician actually do it?"
>
> *Student*: "With a machine."

Attending: "What does the machine, the glucometer, actually do, and what can go wrong?"

The ensuing discussion (which may require an off-rounds visit to the lab) is that most contemporary glucose meters employ an electrochemical method based on classic oxidation–reduction (*redox*) reactions familiar to all medical students and house officers, who may have thought that these concepts were irrelevant to bedside medicine. The gist is that the serum or plasma (the results may differ depending on the source) blood sample is processed such that the glucose is oxidized by an enzyme such as glucose oxidase. The oxidation of glucose leads to a reaction at the electrode, which generates an electrical current. The total charge passing through the electrode is proportional to the amount of glucose in the blood that has reacted with the enzyme.

As a follow-up, you can then inquire: What factors can cause spurious readings? Although laboratory measurements of serum, or preferably plasma, glucose levels are the most accurate, bedside or point-of-care (POC) glucometers are often employed in the hospital to minimize excessive phlebotomy (e.g., in ICUs) when only the glucose level is of interest. The accuracy of different POC glucometers, which use small amounts of whole blood, has been the subject of multiple studies and some debate. Today, U.S. manufacturers must comply with accuracy standards set by the International Organization for Standardization. A glucometer must provide results that are within 20% of the central laboratory standard at least 95% of the time.

Aside from this "baseline" measurement error, comorbid conditions may amplify the error. Anemia has been shown to cause spuriously high readings by POC glucometers because these devices fail to account for reduced plasma displacement by fewer red blood cells, thus artificially elevating the glucose value reported (Figure 3.2). Conversely, patients with polycythemia may have artifactually low readings. Other sources of variability for POC measures include sampling technique, altitude, and ambient temperature.

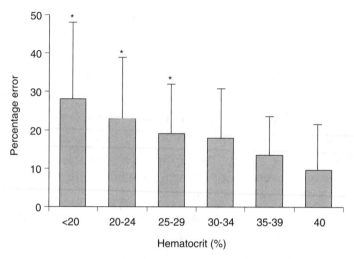

*p<0.001 compared to 40

FIGURE 3.2   Glucometer error. From Mann EA et al. J Diabetes Sci Technol. 2009;3:1319–1329. Reprinted with permission.

MINI-SUMMARY

Common major but avoidable problems related to lab tests are:

- Zigzagging, the inconsistent presentation of findings and the failure to proceed in an orderly way, from noninvasive to invasive. Zigzag presentations are confusing at best and potentially incoherent. This practice may result in serious mistakes.
- Incomplete sourcing and validation of primary data. Never assume that a finding is as reported unless you can validate it.
- Failure to heed the four C's of lab test ordering: contribution, contingency, compliance, and communication.

CHAPTER 4

SEEING IS (ALMOST) BELIEVING: THE IMPORTANCE OF REVIEWING DATA

"Well, now that we *have* seen each other," said the Unicorn, "if you'll believe in me, I'll believe in you. Is that a bargain?" "Yes, if you like," said Alice.

—LEWIS CARROLL (1832–1898)

Seeing is not always believing.

—MARTIN LUTHER KING, JR. (1929–1968)

In medicine we constantly rely on expert interpretations of primary data. We base diagnoses and therapeutic interventions (or noninterventions) on primary sources that we may never see or assess directly. Everyday examples include tissue biopsies, bone marrow aspirates, imaging studies, antinuclear antigen patterns, and cardiac catheterizations. However, just because a report comes from a qualified source does not make it correct. Transcriptional errors or even patient misidentification can render a report inaccurate and misleading. The equipment used to record the test may be malfunctioning or miscalibrated (e.g., assays for measuring prothrombin times).

Becoming a Consummate Clinician: What Every Student, House Officer, and Hospital Practitioner Needs to Know, First Edition.
Ary L. Goldberger and Zachary D. Goldberger.
© 2012 Wiley-Blackwell. Published 2012 by John Wiley & Sons, Inc.

Furthermore, experts can be wrong, either by missing an abnormality or by overcalling one that is not there—examples of the *cognitive errors* described further in Chapter 7. Moreover, when experts disagree, their differences are based largely on the inherent uncertainties and ambiguities in the data. This type of variability is the most difficult for both patients and practitioners to understand and explain. A general and widely held assumption is that the proper tests lead to proper evidence. When you refer a patient for a test or are yourself referred for one, we assume that some answer will be provided and that two experts looking at the data will not hold different and even contradictory perceptions.

However, this expectation is undermined by a fundamental notion: namely, that medical science is built on uncertainty, or, put in other terms, medicine is a probabilistic enterprise. In some cases, the probability of a given diagnosis is essentially 100% (called a *pathognomonic* presentation). Most often, however, the probability is substantially lower. Just as in the quantum microworld of basic physics, uncertainty principles in medicine do not make the science less scientific—instead, uncertainties are woven into the very fabric of the science itself.

UNEXPECTED SOURCES OF VARIABILITY

Inter- and intraobserver variability, even among experts, is an important and often underappreciated source of diagnostic and therapeutic confusion in medicine and sometimes of major medical misjudgments. Interobserver variability means that one interpreter of the data disagrees in part or in full with another. Intraobserver variability means that the same person seeing the same data on different occasions draws different opinions.

Many of the diagnostic decisions we make in medicine are, in large part, influenced by imaging. For example, the presence or absence of an infiltrate on a chest x-ray (CXR) may influence the decision on whether to start antibiotic therapy, sometimes even in the absence of objective signs of infection (e.g., fever, signs of consolidation on chest exam, leukocytosis, sputum findings). We rely heavily on imaging and, more important, the interpretation of these images to help guide our decision making. As such, evaluation of pertinent studies is a key part of clinical presentations.

As introduced in Chapter 3, a huge potential difference exists among the following three statements:

- *The CXR shows a left lower lung field infiltrate.* This statement may imply that you read this study yourself, but is ambiguous with respect to the presenter's connection, if any, to the primary data.
- *The CXR is reported to show a left lower lung field infiltrate.* This implies that some unidentified person read this test and told you the result.
- *The CXR, reviewed with the radiologist, shows a left lower lung field infiltrate.* This statement (the most preferable) implies that you and an expert evaluated the radiograph and discussed the interpretation and differential diagnosis in the context of the patient's presentation.

Students should make it a practice to use the second format when describing data that they have not actually seen. This practice is not a matter of "passing the buck." Rather, it gives the listener a very real sense of the level of confidence in the report and also of the directness of the presenter's contact with the original data. Furthermore, a full understanding of the study in question can be gained by a direct review with the interpreting physician. The bottom-line interpretation says nothing of the thought process that went into the interpretation, nor does it give any indication of the level of uncertainty. Standardized forms for reporting imaging studies often leave little, if any, room for full details.

Medical attendings should, to the extent possible, strive to have their team residents review all studies of consequence with an expert. Other options would be to devote 15 minutes of rounds to the radiology suite, pathology lab, or echocardiogram reading room. Any editorial comment that can be made about the official reading is often very helpful. Also be aware that abnormalities present on a given imaging study may belie the degree of illness seen at the bedside. For example, consider a 40-year-old man who presents with new-onset heart failure with a globally reduced, left ventricular ejection fraction of 30% by echocardiogram. However, his coronary angiogram shows only a 70% mid-left anterior descending stenosis. The latter finding is not sufficient to explain the severe degree of heart failure seen; a diagnosis of "ischemic cardiomyopathy" would at best be incomplete, and probably entirely incorrect.

ASSESSING OBSERVER VARIABILITY

The medical literature is replete with studies documenting inter- and intraobserver variability. Notable examples come from the interpretation of screening mammograms, pulmonary CT scans for nodules, and pathology specimens such as cervical biopsies. For example, Figure 4.1 (interobserver) shows the sometimes wide and surprising

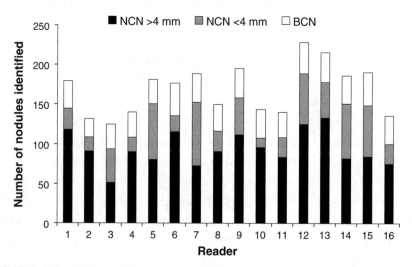

FIGURE 4.1 When different experts look at the same data. Bar graphs of diagnostic frequencies for individual pulmonary CT scan readers show considerable interobserver variability in final case diagnosis and number of nodules recorded among different readers. BCN, benign calcified nodule; NCN, noncalcified nodule. Particularly surprising are the discrepancies in the identification by expert radiologists of large noncalcified nodules. (From Gierada DS, et al. Interobserver agreement on interpretation of pulmonary findings at low-dose CT screening. Radiology. 2008;246:265–272. Reprinted with permission.)

TABLE 4.1 Kappa Statistic

Kappa Value	Interpretation
0–0.2	Slight agreement between observers
0.21–0.4	Fair agreement between observers
0.41–0.6	Moderate agreement between observers
0.61–0.8	Substantial agreement between observers
0.81–1.0	Almost perfect agreement between observers

discrepancies among 16 radiologists from the 10 National Lung Screening Trial screening centers of the National Cancer Institute's Lung Screening Study network who reviewed image subsets from 135 baseline low-dose screening chest CT examinations.

A variety of statistical tests have been devised to measure inter- and intraobserver variability. One frequently used statistic is *kappa*, a measure of how often two observers agree compared with chance (Table 4.1). A number of implementations of the kappa statistic have been proposed. However, you need to exercise caution in interpreting studies purporting to test for observer variability since three key issues may *not* be reported:

1. How often do multiple expert observers agree with each other? What is their degree of *concordance*?
2. What is the range of interexpert agreement with a gold standard of merit for both pathological and control tissue samples or images? What is the *accuracy*? Keep in mind that such a gold standard may not exist or whether it exists may itself be the subject of debate.
3. What is the percentage, with confidence intervals, of *major* disagreements—those actually affecting management?

Simple agreement on whether a biopsy or an image study represents health or disease is not sufficiently informative. The degree of agreement with respect to the type of disease (e.g., class of lymphoma) and extent (e.g., whether or not there is local spread of a prostate tumor) is also of vital importance. Inter- and intraobserver variability is most impactful when the discrepancies will alter management plans: the decision to treat and, if so, what the optimal therapeutic options would be. In the study described above, the report of a large noncalcified nodule vs. a benign calcified nodule will probably lead to very different diagnostic and therapeutic approaches.

As another example, suppose that during rounds you are surprised by the apparent amount of variability you encounter in the way in which house officers report the grade of cardiac murmurs. These discrepancies motivate you to consider conducting a more formal, prospective study of detection and gradation of murmurs by interns and residents. You think about adding a comparison with a trained observer, a cardiologist who is blinded to echocardiographic findings done on this admission. However, disagreements about whether an aortic outflow murmur is grade I or II vs. III (soft vs. relatively loud) are inconsequential if no change in workup or treatment would be affected. On the other hand, if the disparities were associated with a missed diagnosis of critical aortic stenosis, the variability would have a profound impact on decision making.

Study design and statistical analysis should be geared to addressing these issues of clinical impact, not just quantifying observer variability. In this example, beyond the gradation of the murmur, the key clinical question is whether the patient has none or mild, moderate, or severe aortic stenosis. Your study design would then need to be enlarged to include vital signs, carotid pulse assessment, and left ventricular impulse palpation.

COMPUTER INTERPRETATIONS

Modern medicine is unimaginable without digital computing. One question central to the artificial intelligence community is whether— in addition to data preprocessing, processing, and storage—computers can also replace or even improve on human interpretations of certain clinical tests that are based on image or waveform analysis. Computer analysis of CBCs is routine in a Coulter counter but does not replace human oversight in studies flagged as unusual.

What about reading x-rays or ECGs? The latter would appear to be particularly suitable for full-scale automation given the fact that diagnoses are based on waveform recordings in only 12 leads (related to electrode configurations). In fact, most contemporary ECG machines provide a computerized interpretation option. Although interpretation software in the electrocardiograph is improving, the accuracy of these digital analyses is fraught with error. Further, the more abnormal the recording, the greater the likelihood that the computer will make mistakes of consequence (e.g., missing atrial fibrillation or calling it present when it is not). From a clinical point of view, computer ECG readings are helpful in guiding clinicians and sometimes in pointing out findings otherwise overlooked. However, computer-generated reports should always be taken with a proverbial grain of salt and considered preliminary at best, and often entirely or partially wrong.

Dr. David Spodick and colleagues at the University of Massachusetts Medical School surprisingly found that computers were also susceptible to intraobserver variability. Two clinically identical ECGs from the same patient obtained minutes apart were read by a computer program. The computer readings sometimes showed major differences in interpretation in the absence of any clinical change apparent to an expert. The source of this unanticipated "computer intraobserver" variability is not clear, but the consequences could be substantial. Dr. Spodick aptly called this phenomenon *computer treason*. However, the real crime may be human overestimation of the abilities and underestimation of the limitations of computational devices.

COPING WITH OBSERVER VARIABILITY

Many students and even senior clinicians are surprised by the amount of observer variability (human or computer) in interpreting certain tests that they rely on heavily for key management decisions. Patients and their families are even more surprised and probably assume that the interpretation of medical tests is consistent and reliable. Here are five practical recommendations for *evidence-based* assessment of test results for students and house officers:

1. For major tests affecting management, you should make an effort to assess the reliability of the test (false positives and false negatives) and observer variability based on a critical look at the literature.
2. Wherever possible, review the primary data with an expert.
3. In presentations, indicate whether or not you have seen key observable data and what or who is the source of the interpretation.
4. If feasible, *re-look* at the same data with another expert to see if the interpretations are the same. (Happily, the vast majority of specialists enjoy scientific discussions of observer variability and reviewing findings with students. Reports of medical student defenestrations during such "second opinion" requests are purely anecdotal and are probably overestimated.)
5. Never rely on automated (computer) assessments for definitive diagnoses. This advice is particularly relevant for ECG interpretations, as machine readings are widely disseminated but sometimes fail to get critically reviewed.

Note to Attendings. Attendings are always trying to assess the validity of data that are presented to them by members of the rounding team. A strategy for both teaching and learning about the limits of reliability is to interrupt presentations of test results and ask what the sensitivity and specificity of a given finding are for some condition, what populations were used to obtain these numbers, and if there is information on observer variability. Whenever a team member answers a question (e.g., about sensitivity, specificity, left ventricular ejection fraction) with a hard number such as "30%," the follow-up should be: What are the confidence intervals around that number, the "error bars" that that we expect with all other scientific types of point estimates (e.g., relative risks, odds ratios, mean and median values)? If a review of the literature does not permit such an assessment, that information is also valuable. A better way to state the statistic would be that the "reported sensitivity of this test is relatively low, estimated to be about 30%."

A RELATED CAUTION: CUT-AND-PASTE WORKUPS

We live in an increasingly digital world. One advantage is the ready access to and transmissibility of electronic medical data such as blood test reports and imaging studies. However, the ability to literally "grab" such data and paste them into medical write-ups must be done with great caution, as the information may be incomplete or inaccurate. Errors that get embedded in the record this way may get propagated through countless cycles of cutting and pasting. Such "mutations" can at least be sources of confusion. In the worst-case scenarios, they may be lethal if they include information that is incomplete or inaccurate. Or they may lead to major errors in treatment if not updated as illustrated in the example. Make sure that you evaluate all the data you enter into a record and always be on the lookout for inconsistencies or data that require updating.

EXAMPLE: CUT-AND-PASTE PERILS

Mrs. Grimm, an 85-year-old woman, was admitted to the intensive care unit with acute respiratory distress syndrome due to Streptococcus pneumoniae bacteremia. She was intubated, requiring 100% oxygen to maintain a PaO_2 above 90 mmHg, and her condition was not improving, despite supportive care and broad-spectrum antibiotic therapy. Although her family members, at the bedside daily, were initially hopeful about the possibility of recovery, the discussion of her poor prognosis was addressed each day by the members of the ICU team and the palliative care team. The intern was present during all of these discussions and was careful to document the patient's "full code" status in the note.

After five days without improvement, and progressive hypotension necessitating increasing doses of dopamine, the family reported to the team after rounds that in concordance with the patient's previously expressed wishes, they wanted no resuscitative efforts in the event of cardiopulmonary arrest. Her code status was changed to DNR (do not resuscitate). The resident, not present on rounds in the morning, wrote the note. Aware only of her critically ill yet relatively unchanged clinical status, he updated the electronic note with the new labs and vital signs but kept the rest of the note the same, including her previous full code status.

At midnight, the patient went into a pulseless electrical activity (PEA) arrest, and the code team was called. The intern on the code team was asked to quickly read the most recent progress note and give the code leader an impression of the patient and the code status. Maximum-dose vasopressors were initiated, and after several unsuccessful attempts at additional central venous access and 45 minutes of chest compressions, resulting in numerous rib fractures, the patient expired. Only after the prolonged resuscitation was it learned that the patient was made DNR that morning. The patient's husband was called after the code, and asked what happened.

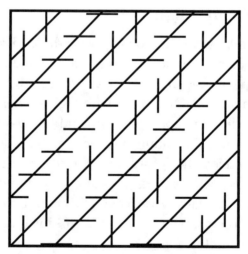

FIGURE 4.2   The Zoellner illusion. Are the longer lines parallel?

FINAL NOTE: WHEN SEEING AND BELIEVING DIVERGE

The discussion in this chapter has emphasized the visual review of data. Literally looking at data yourself with an expert who is not biased by other clinical data is always recommended, particularly when the interpretation will have an important impact on decision making. However, as indicated in the opening quotes of this chapter, the adage that "seeing is believing" is an oversimplification if taken too literally. We can easily be misled by any of our senses and a radiologist may convince us of a finding that is not clearly present. The limitations of visual assessment are nicely illustrated in a famous visual trick, the Zoellner illusion (Figure 4.2). The long lines are actually parallel. But the crossed lines create the impression that these long tracks are going to intersect. They never will but our eyes suggest otherwise. So seeing is (almost) believing in the sense that clinicians, like Pulitzer Prize journalists and historians, need to source their data and, whenever possible, review it with an expert or two, especially if the findings are ambiguous.

CHAPTER 5

"WORSTS FIRST": HOW TO FRAME A DIFFERENTIAL DIAGNOSIS

Art consists of limitation. The most beautiful part of every picture is the frame.

—GILBERT K. CHESTERTON (1874–1936)

Clinical decision making is distinct from that of virtually every other type of profession. At least two ingredients make it unique. One is that clinicians almost always base their assessments on physical contact with the patient. Second, experienced clinicians, at least subliminally, implement a *two-tiered* analytic process in framing a differential diagnosis of what is wrong with a given patient, which can be described as a bit like the classic London double-decker sightseeing bus. The first tier is based on the principle of *worsts first*—the urgent consideration of all the possible diagnoses that might literally kill someone and need to be excluded right away, regardless of their statistical rarity. The second tier is a more comprehensive list of considerations—the set of all or most of the possible causes of the patient's problems, including both rarer and more common conditions. The latter can be viewed as the "all things considered" category. To illustrate this two-tiered approach, we selected the differential diagnosis of two of the most common and important presenting

Becoming a Consummate Clinician: What Every Student, House Officer, and Hospital Practitioner Needs to Know, First Edition.
Ary L. Goldberger and Zachary D. Goldberger.

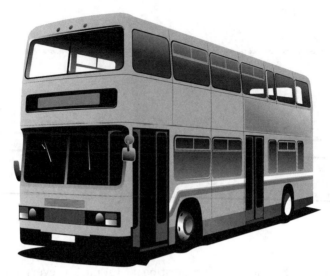

Double-decker bus as a metaphor for two-tiered thinking.

symptoms in clinical and emergency medicine: chest discomfort and right upper quadrant pain.

DIFFERENTIAL DIAGNOSIS OF CHEST DISCOMFORT

Chest Discomfort: Worsts First

There are multiple causes of chest discomfort (this problem is usually considered under the heading *chest pain*). However, patients with acute or chronic coronary syndromes—stable or unstable angina and even acute myocardial infarction—often emphatically deny having *pain* but will admit to having chest *discomfort or chest "pressure."* Of these causes, only a handful of diagnoses are both life-threatening and treatable in the immediate term and, therefore, need to be considered urgently and excluded. These potentially lethal causes of chest discomfort (pain) can be grouped into three categories: cardiovascular, pleuropulmonary, and gastrointestinal (Exhibit 5.1).

1. *Cardiovascular causes of chest discomfort* include (a) acute coronary syndromes, (b) aortic aneurysms (dissecting or expanding), and (c) acute pericarditis. Of these, acute pericarditis

EXHIBIT 5.1   Major, Life-Threatening Causes of Chest Discomfort: Worsts First

Cardiovascular
  Acute coronary (ischemic) syndromes, including Takotsubo cardiomyopathy
  Aortic aneurysm (dissecting or expanding)
  Pericarditis, especially with effusion
  Severe aortic stenosis
  Myocarditis
Pleuropulmonary
  Acute pulmonary embolus
  Pneumonitis syndromes
  Pneumothorax
Gastrointestinal
  Ruptured esophagus
  Gastric–duodenal ulcers, especially with bleeding or rupture
  Acute pancreatobiliary syndromes

is the least likely to be fatal but needs to be among those considered first because it (a) can lead to death from cardiac tamponade if an effusion is present, (b) is a contraindication to anticoagulation, and (c) may be associated with other life-threatening conditions, such as systemic lupus erythematosus and chronic renal failure—and in the case of an effusion due to malignancy.

2. *Pleuropulmonary causes of chest discomfort*, often but not always with dyspnea, include (a) pulmonary embolism, (b) pneumothorax, and (c) pneumonia.

3. *Gastrointestinal causes of chest discomfort* can be subgrouped into those originating above or below the diaphragm. In the former category is one major condition: (a) ruptured esophagus (Boerhaave's syndrome). In the latter category are (b) gastroduodenal ulcers and (c) acute pancreatobiliary disease (primarily acute pancreatitis and/or cholecystitis). One (or, occasionally, a combination) of these potentially life-threatening conditions should always be considered in every patient presenting with chest pain/discomfort. Obviously, not every cause can be ruled out. There is a key difference between formulating a differential and testing for the components in the differential. Clinical

acumen must always guide the most appropriate workup based on limited history and emergency department physical, under pressured circumstances.

The need to consider life-threatening causes (*worsts first*) is not meant to imply that every imaging and diagnostic technique available is to be used in every case. Consideration of worsts first is indicated as a cognitive reflex, not as a prescription to order tests as part of defensive medicine. A strong knowledge base coupled with careful history and physical exams remain the best antidotes to what Dr. Pat Croskerry has termed *base rate neglect*. Under this rubric, he includes the tendency to inflate the actual prevalence of a disease to avoid missing rare but life-threatening illnesses. In addition, the initial workup by the emergency department should be discussed in a critical but positive way to learn the basis on which certain conditions were ruled out or ruled in.

Note to Attendings. When hearing a presentation of a patient admitted via the emergency department, a useful exercise is to *freeze-frame* the presentation at selected points to ask the ward team: What would you have done at this point? What options were available? This strategy encourages active listening, creates suspense, and most important, compels a critical assessment of the workup in real time.

Chest Discomfort: All Things Considered

Sometimes the initial assessment of chest discomfort does not uncover a definitive cause and, most important, does not reveal evidence of one of the major life-threatening conditions noted above. In such instances it is helpful to take a step back and consider the more general set of conditions that may be associated with chest discomfort. This lengthier (but still not complete) list is summarized in Exhibit 5.2 and obviously includes all of the conditions mentioned above.

A useful strategy for thinking about the global differential diagnosis of chest discomfort—more reliable than most mnemonic

EXHIBIT 5.2   More Comprehensive Differential Diagnosis of Chest Pain: "Onion Skin" or "Mental Body Scan" Approach

Dermatologic
   Herpes zoster (involving a left chest dermatome)
Psychiatric
   Panic/anxiety attack
   Munchausen's syndrome
Musculoskeletal
   Muscle strain
   Costochondritis (Tietze's syndrome)
   Rib bruise or fracture
Neural Compressive
   Cervical radiculitis
   Vertebral compression fracture
Pleuropulmonary
   Acute pulmonary embolus
   Pneumonitis syndromes
   Pneumothorax
   Tumor
Cardiovascular
   Acute coronary (ischemic) syndromes[a]
   Aortic aneurysm (dissecting or expanding)
   Pericarditis
   Aortic stenosis
   Myocarditis
Gastrointestinal
   Esophageal
   Esophagitis/reflux
   Esophageal dysmotility syndromes/spasm
   Ruptured esophagus
   Gastroduodenal ulcers, malignant or nonmalignant
   Gastritis
Acute Pancreatobiliary Syndromes
   Acute or recurrent pancreatitis
   Acute cholecystitis

[a]Includes other nonatherosclerotic causes of infarction/ischemia, such as collagen vascular disease, coronary artery dissection, coronary artery spasm syndromes (Prinzmetal's angina/variant angina), takotsubo (stress) cardiomyopathy, cocaine-related, and congenital heart disease (e.g., anomalous left circumflex artery).

devices—is to work your way from the outside of the body inward in concentric rings (*onion skinning or mental body scanning*) and from head downward. The causes can include everything from left-sided dermatomal discomfort with herpes zoster, to cervical disk disease with radicular pain, to vertebral compression fractures with radiation of pain in an anterior direction.

An understandable and universal goal in crafting differential diagnoses is being comprehensive and crisp, in the mode of the *New England Journal of Medicine's* (*NEJM's*) Clinicopathologic Conferences (CPCs) or its Clinical Problem-Solving (CPS) cases. In the best of these cases, the discussant deftly delineates and distinguishes among a myriad of possibilities and seems, with magical finesse, to hone in on the correct diagnosis with the sharpness of Ockham's razor (Chapter 8). It is an admirable model, much envied but much less often achieved in the hurly-burly of the real world, where cases play out prospectively and are not written up "after the fact" and where more than one diagnosis may be present.

Indeed, the success of the discussants of CPCs or CPS cases in the *NEJM* and other journals is remarkable and primarily a testament to the extraordinary diagnostic skills of these master clinicians. But keep in mind that these discussants are operating in a rather specialized arena where cases are handpicked based on their discussant's expertise, the cases' uniqueness, and also because these cases have definitive answers supported by "smoking gun" evidence, typically from biopsies or postmortem studies. The revelatory climax is often preceded by the phrase: "A procedure was done. . . ." Then we learn that the heart failure was due to Chagas disease (American trypanosomiasis) or the splenomegaly and fever to visceral leishmaniasis contracted on a recreational trip to Central America, or the mid-right lower abdominal pain was due to carcinoid and not to appendicitis. Indeed, heart failure due to Chagas disease is much more likely to show up in a case report than in your clinic practice in North America. Similarly, the Bayesian probabilities in the emergency department or ICU, where "all-comer" cases are self-presented, are very different from the pretest likelihoods in a highly selected CPC/CPS forum.

DIFFERENTIAL DIAGNOSIS OF RIGHT UPPER QUADRANT PAIN

As with chest pain, there are many causes of right upper quadrant (RUQ) pain, and this complaint comprises only a subset of the causes of abdominal pain. Similar to chest pain, only a few are both life-threatening and treatable in the immediate term. As with chest pain, begin with anatomy: hepatobiliary system, duodenum, pancreas, right kidney, mesenteric vessels, right hemidiaphragm, and right lower lung lobe. Next, consider the possible causes in terms of pathology (i.e., vascular, inflammatory, neoplastic, traumatic, etc.). An abdominal exam is essential in trying to elucidate a cause (e.g., rebound tenderness, bowel sounds, guarding). Exhibit 5.3 is a short list of treatable "worsts firsts." A more exhaustive list is given in Exhibit 5.4

EXHIBIT 5.3   Major Life-Threatening Causes of RUQ Pain: Worsts Firsts

Hepatobiliary	Hepatitis syndromes
	Hepatic abscess
	Liver tumors
	Hepatic congestion syndromes:
	Severe heart failure
	Budd–Chiari syndrome
	Cholecystitis/choledocholithiasis/cholangitis
Gastroduodenal	Penetrating ulcer
Pancreatic	Pancreatitis
	Pancreatic cancer
Right renal	Pyelonephritis
	Stones
	Renal vein thrombosis
	Tumor
Right colonic	Diverticulitis
	Tumor
	Volvulus or other obstructive lesion
	Gallstone ileus
Diaphragmatic	Tear
	Abscess
Lymphatic	Lymphoma
Right pleuropulmonary	Effusion/pleurisy
	Pulmonary embolism
	Right lower lobe infection or tumor

EXHIBIT 5.4 Life-Threatening Causes of RUQ Pain: A More Comprehensive List[a]

Dermatologic
  Herpes zoster (involving a lower right chest or upper right abdomen dermatome)
  Cellulitis
Musculoskeletal
  Muscle strain
Diaphragmatic
  Ventral/incisional/para-esophageal hernia
  Diaphragmatic abscess
Hepatic
  Contusion
  Abscess
  Hepatic congestion (right heart failure or hepatic vein thrombosis:
    Budd–Chiari syndrome)
  Hepatitis syndrome
  Infarction
  Tumors: benign and malignant
Biliary
  Choledocholithiasis
  Cholangitis
  Cholecystitis
  Tumors
  Traumatic rupture
Duodenal
  Ulcer (penetrating; nonpenetrating)
  Duodenitis
  Obstruction
  Post-ERCP duodenal perforation related to sphincterotomy
Right colonic
  Diverticulitis
  Colitis
  Obstruction: tumor, volvulus or other obstructive lesion, gallstone ileus
Right renal
  Pyelonephritis
  Renal infarct
  Renal–ureteral calculus
  Renal vein thrombosis
  Renal tumor
Lymphatic
  Lymphoma
Pancreatic
  Pancreatitis
  Pancreatic carcinoma
  Pancreatic cyst
Vascular
  Mesenteric arterial thrombosis or embolism

---

[a]In addition, consider rarer causes, such as thoracic spine pathology (multiple myeloma, metastases, osteoarthritis with vertebral compression, tuberculosis, rheumatoid spondylitis) and adrenal gland pathology [Waterhouse–Friderichsen syndrome (hemorrhagic adrenalitis), neuroblastoma, adrenal infarct].

"*n*-PLUS": A FINAL NOTE ON CRAFTING DIFFERENTIAL DIAGNOSES

You should always consider every differential diagnosis to be "*n plus*," where *n* is the sum of all the things you are considering and *plus* is the possibility of other alternative(s). The latter most often is something that you had not thought of at the time. Yet sometimes, in very special cases, it is something entirely new—the discovery of a novel syndrome. More often it is a somewhat off-beat or unexpected presentation of a well-known disease process, or a true *forme fruste* (highly atypical or incomplete presentation of a known disease, from the French for "incomplete form"). The "*n* plus" rule is an example of what some authors refer to more generically as "lateral thinking" or "thinking outside the box." We prefer *n plus* since you can actually add a written or at least a mental line on the differential diagnosis to "Consider other possibilities," making this an explicit rather than an implicit part of clinical evaluation.

EXAMPLE

An otherwise healthy 53-year-old man with a history of aortic insufficiency who was 20 years status post a mechanical prosthetic aortic valve replacement presented with high fevers and left shoulder pain. The obvious concerns included bacterial endocarditis with arthropathy and/or a primary septic joint or septic shoulder bursitis. Physical examination, initial laboratory studies, including a transesophageal echocardiogram with particular attention to the prosthetic aortic valve, and blood cultures were unrevealing. About 36 hours after hospital admission, with hydration, a community-acquired left lower lobe pneumonia with referred pain to the left shoulder became apparent.

Suggested Exercise

Try constructing two-tiered differential diagnoses of some other major symptoms and signs and compare notes with your colleagues and attendings. Some common acute differentials include fever, weight loss, headache, red eye, acute visual loss, epigastric pain, shortness of breath, diarrhea, weakness, and selected electrolyte disorders, among others.

As with lab tests, expecting the unexpected is a principle that applies to formulating a differential diagnosis. While worsts first and a subsequent onion peel-back approach is a good systematic way to narrow your differential, revisiting unexpected causes, as in the example above, is often enormously helpful.

Sir Arthur Conan Doyle is best known as the author and creator of the Sherlock Holmes series. Conan Doyle was also a physician who reportedly modeled his protagonist's deductive reasoning skills on one of his own professors at the University of Edinburgh, Dr. Joseph Bell.

One of the Sherlock Holmes stories, "Silver Blaze," features the disappearance of a famous horse before an important race, and the apparent murder of its trainer. The following interchange between Holmes and a Scotland Yard detective, Inspector Gregory, illustrates how what does not happen can be as important as what does.

> *Gregory*: Is there any other point to which you would wish to draw my attention?
> *Holmes*: To the curious incident of the dog in the night-time.
> *Gregory*: The dog did nothing in the night-time.
> *Holmes*: That was the curious incident.

MINI-SUMMARY

- Differential diagnosis can be approached in a two-tiered way. First, rule out (or in) diagnoses that could be lethal or lead to major harm if not recognized promptly. Second, if none of these diagnoses is apparent, step back and take a more comprehensive view, organized anatomically or physiologically, allowing a type of "body scan."
- Adopt the *n* plus rule: You should always consider every differential diagnosis to be *n plus*, where *n* is the sum of all the things you are considering and plus is the possibility of some other alternative(s).

CHAPTER 6

CLINICAL QUERIES: ASKING THE 3½ KEY QUESTIONS

It is better to know some of the questions than all of the answers.
—JAMES THURBER (1894–1961)

We live in a "bottom-line" culture. The need for multitasking during rounds creates additional pressures to "get to the point." The more urgent the situation, the greater the pressures are to fast-track to those action points. At the same time, clinical decision making is replete with ambiguities, false starts, false positives, and false negatives. Life and trying to keep people alive are complex enterprises. The way we frame questions, just as the way we frame images, is often a key to what we see or don't see.

GLIMPSE VS. GAZE: WHAT THINKING MODE TO PRESCRIBE ON THE WARDS

Clinicians resemble major league baseball hitters, who face a daunting array of tough pitchers (our patients) who throw a lot of curveballs and change-ups. But unlike major leaguers, who can win batting titles by *not* getting a hit in two of three chances (i.e., batting ".333"),

Becoming a Consummate Clinician: What Every Student, House Officer, and Hospital Practitioner Needs to Know, First Edition.
Ary L. Goldberger and Zachary D. Goldberger.

clinicians must try to bat "1.000" Like good hitters, experienced clinicians learn to "look for pitches" and to think primarily about one or two main possibilities when they hear about a case. Developing an *anticipatory intuition* or *framework* is essential in clinical medicine. A related part of clinical diagnostic skills is the ability to assess a situation and make correct diagnoses within seconds or minutes of hearing or seeing a case. The ability to *size things up* is especially important in acute settings such as the emergency department, intensive and critical care situations, and in surgical and other procedure suites.

This type of intuitive sensibility is related to the well-known phenomenon of the validity of first impressions. Author Malcolm Gladwell describes and celebrates this phenomenon of intuition in his provocative 2005 book, *Blink: The Power of Thinking Without Thinking*. As Gladwell notes: "There can be as much value in the blink of an eye as in months of rational analysis."

Leaps of intuition are not magical, but they are still neurophysiologically mysterious. Perhaps these "aha" moments have to do with the brain's nonlinear capacity to integrate past experience and process multiple cues and clues. Test takers, including those grappling with the Medical College Admission Test, medical boards, and certification maintenance examinations, often apply this principle, which is the basis of the adage "When in doubt, go with your first impression."

In the contemporary language of complex systems, an intuitive insight is an example of an *emergent process in which the entire thought or insight cannot be reduced to a simple addition of its components.* Intuitions are the "eureka moments" of life and an essential feature not only of our daily, creative functioning but also of clinical reasoning. In this respect, creative intuition is not at all like a kaleidoscopic image, where the pieces all add up to the final design. Instead, emergent ideas are more like the nonlinear creation of the Mandelbrot set, a fractal object that seems to explode from a deceptively simple recipe (Figure 6.1).

Yet intuitions can also be wildly off base, to use another baseball metaphor, and constitute only one component of clinical assessment, which must be carefully validated and tested. Thus, a key skill to develop so as not to miss diagnoses is the complementary and

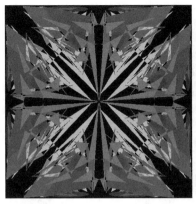 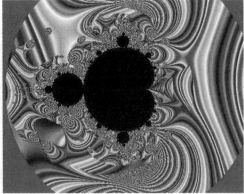

FIGURE 6.1   Kaleidoscopic image (left panel, a linear object) vs. the Mandelbrot fractal set (right panel, a nonlinear object). Which is more complex?

essential ability to consider all of the other possibilities when thinking about diagnosis, etiology, and therapy. Sometimes our first impressions—the blinks—are dreadfully wrong or, at the very best or least, incomplete.

Dr. Jerome Groopman at Harvard Medical School has written eloquently about this competing challenge between intuition and reflection in his book *How Doctors Think*. As noted by Dr. Groopman: "Doctors must be wary of 'going with your gut' when what's in your gut is a strong emotion about a patient, even a positive one. This species of 'affective bias' can skew a physician's judgment and lead to misdiagnoses."

Another mechanism of misdiagnosis has been called *confirmation bias* or *anchoring*. As Dr. Groopman explains: "Anchoring is a shortcut in thinking where a person doesn't consider multiple possibilities but quickly and firmly latches on to a single one, sure that he has thrown his anchor down just where he needs to be." Clinicians therefore need to cultivate an approach that incorporates simultaneously two tendencies that are seemingly at odds with each other: intuition and systematic thinking. This competition could be referred to as the *glimpse* vs. the *gaze*.

In actuality, this either–or distinction is itself an oversimplification. In addition to quick and longer looks, clinicians need to cultivate a third modality of seeing: the *re-look*—the self-imposed intellectual discipline to revisit first, second, and even third impressions and to be open to the "possibility of other possibilities." In medicine, these other possibilities include diagnoses not yet considered and, in rare but path-breaking cases, new syndromes and diseases that remain to be discovered, or novel presentations of known pathologies.

Keep in mind that not too long ago the first recognized cases of HIV/AIDS, severe acute respiratory syndrome (SARS), and the Brugada syndrome were reported. One of the most exciting facets of clinical medicine is that the next patient you admit to your service or see in the clinic might fall into the latter group of about-to-be-recognized diseases or reportable presentations. Most exciting is that such discoveries are as open to medical students as they are to seasoned clinicians.

Finally, as noted by Dr. Groopman:

> A technique to foster this type of critical thinking is for clinicians to develop a routine, much like they prescribe for exercise protocols. The idea of a routine here is not intended to foster a reflexive type of predictability. Rather, it is intended to encourage "out of the box" thinking by opening up the number of options being considered, and by encouraging the search for alternative explanations.

THE 3½ KEY QUESTIONS RULE

From a practical point of view, how can you combine the glimpse and the gaze: to be both intuitive and expeditious but also thoughtful and comprehensive? Obviously, there is no single "mechanism" to achieve this aim. But for most situations in clinical medicine, especially involving diagnostic considerations, and applicable when looking at clinical data sets (e.g., lab test results) or physiologic recording studies (e.g., ECG), it is worth asking the *3½ key questions*:

- What is it, and what else could it be (Dx and DDx)?
- What factor(s) could have caused it (etiology)?
- What are the therapeutic options (Rx/Tx)?

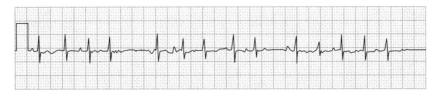

FIGURE 6.2   An irregular rhythm. Compare and contrast with Figure 6.3.

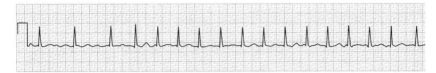

FIGURE 6.3   Your patient's ECG (lead II) shows an irregular rhythm. What is the diagnosis? What is the differential diagnosis?

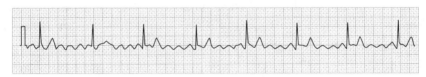

FIGURE 6.4   This rhythm strip resembles atrial fibrillation but is actually due to something else.

To illustrate this approach, let's begin with an example from ECG analysis (Figures 6.2 to 6.4). Beyond its utility as a vital clinical skill, ECG interpretation is important because it exemplifies and reinforces the universal clinical needs to be both systematic and thorough. Consider the ECG of a patient with palpitations shown in Figure 6.2. The lead II rhythm strip shows a rapid irregular rhythm with a narrow QRS complex. If you describe this over the phone to a colleague or look at it in the usual clinical haste, atrial fibrillation will probably be the initial "blink" impression, leading to anticoagulation, antiarrhythmic therapy, and possible consideration of electrical) cardioversion.

Taking a step back and looking at the differential diagnosis (DDx) of a *rapid and irregular narrow complex (normal QRS duration) rhythm* is a useful exercise. The DDx includes not only atrial fibrillation but four other major possibilities:

1. Atrial flutter with a variable ventricular response
2. Multifocal atrial tachycardia (MAT)
3. Sinus tachycardia with frequent atrial premature complexes
4. Artifact simulating atrial fibrillation, usually due to a noisy baseline or sometimes to tremor, as in Parkinson's disease. The muscle tremor may "contaminate" the ECG, giving the full impression of a cardiac arrhythmia.

A closer look at the rhythm strip in question reveals that it is actually MAT, a rhythm that simulates atrial fibrillation but has quite distinct etiological implications and management. MAT is defined by the appearance of three or more consecutive nonsinus P waves at a rapid rate. The most common substrates are chronic obstructive pulmonary disease (COPD), usually with an acute or subacute exacerbation, or severe organic heart disease. The management of MAT in COPD entails therapy of the underlying pulmonary process and sometimes use of calcium channel blockers such as diltiazem for rate control. However, in contrast to atrial fibrillation, MAT is *not* an indication for anticoagulation (unless it leads to or is associated with atrial fibrillation). Further, electrical cardioversion for MAT will be ineffective and potentially hazardous. For contrast and comparison, an example of actual atrial fibrillation is shown in Figure 6.3.

For additional comparison, the third ECG case (Figure 6.4) indicates the complications in differential diagnosis introduced by artifact—spurious findings that simulate medical diagnoses and that often lead clinicians astray. In this case, artifact gives the appearance of atrial flutter or fibrillation in a patient with coronary artery disease who is actually in sinus rhythm.

These examples illustrate the problems of relying on the blink reflex to make clinical assessments. The pitfalls of overreliance on initial intuitions are also illustrated by an example (Figure 6.5) from a setting that would appear to have no relation to clinical medicine.

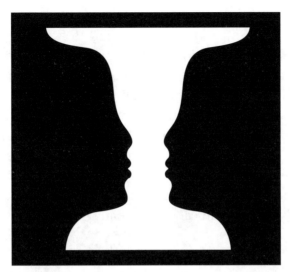

FIGURE 6.5 What do you see in this simple-appearing black-and-white image?

This black-and-white drawing is an optical illusion that you have probably seen—but not in medical school. It is sometimes called the *Rubin Vase* after the Dutch psychologist Edgar Rubin, who made these images famous.

Take a quick look (blink or glimpse). What do you see? A vase (white central area) or two faces (black side areas)? Different observers have different first impressions. But with further attention (gazing), the flickering of this picture between the two images is apparent. Furthermore, what we first see may be biased by what we are told to look for: one vase or two faces. This type of expectational bias as a source of medical errors is discussed further in Chapter 7.

This illusion is also medically relevant (in case you were still puzzled) because it illustrates the clinical principle that a single impression may at best be only partly insightful or explanatory. Further scrutiny yields additional information and raises additional questions. The illusion illustrates symbolically that in medicine, as in art, more than one meaning or diagnosis may be at play simultaneously. Patients not infrequently present with two or more concomitant conditions, which may or may not be directly related.

EXAMPLE

A 79-year-old man complained of fatigue. He was found to be hypo-kalemic with increased urinary K^+ concentration. CBC and other relevant tests were normal. Abdominal imaging studies revealed an adrenal mass consistent with an adenoma, and the presumptive diagnosis of Conn's syndrome (primary hyperaldosteronism) was made. However, K^+ repletion and treatment with amiloride failed to fully relieve his symptoms. He also had unexplained splenomegaly. A few years later he presented with chronic granulocytic leukemia, which was probably in a preclinical state initially.

Sometimes, identifying one explanatory diagnosis may mask another or inhibit the search for even more alternatives—the "case is solved" syndrome of anchoring. In the example above, the diagnosis of Conn's syndrome seemed to nail down the cause of the patient's fatigue. However, another diagnosis, chronic granulocytic leukemia, was lurking in the background. Understandably, there is the human reaction that "one explanatory diagnosis is enough, so let's not go looking for trouble."

Dual or multiple diagnoses have major implications only if the conditions are treatable. In the latter category would be a patient presenting with heart failure and known hypertension and coronary artery disease who has developed critical aortic stenosis, a surgically remediable lesion. Not asking "What else could be causing the heart failure—beyond hypertension and coronary disease?" would have profound implications for aortic valve replacement, a potentially life-saving intervention.

Learning and practicing critical thinking skills that resist conventional wisdom, actively looking for anomalous findings, and harnessing the energies of imagination are powerful antidotes to cognitive errors (Chapter 7). From a more positive perspective, critical and imaginative thinking are the sources of successful therapeutic interventions and clinical discoveries. As noted above, perhaps one of the patients you are seeing now has a new syndrome yet to be recognized.

Helping trainees acquire and master these skills that join the systematic with the imaginative is one of the most challenging educational goals in medicine, particularly in this age of distracting info-glut (see the Introduction).

BEYOND THE 3½ KEY QUESTIONS

These practical questions are intended to provide an orienting space to explore clinical possibilities, with particular emphasis on always asking "What else could it be?" as a cognitive reflex and of considering the widest range of therapeutic options. However, trainees and their mentors should be mindful that the very act of posing essential queries may squeeze out other important questions that then remain unasked. For example, a major limitation of the *Dx/Rx–Cause(s)–Therapeutic Options* paradigm is that it does not explicitly address mechanisms of disease, the deeper understanding of the physiological and pathophysiological processes that underlie diagnostic considerations. Getting at these deeper issues is metaphorically like peeling back the next layer of the onion, which in the parlance of critical thinking is sometimes termed the transition from *information* and *knowledge* to *understanding*.

In the case presented above of MAT vs. atrial fibrillation, this deeper probing leads to the frontiers of clinical cardiac electrophysiology. The mechanisms of these arrhythmias are only incompletely understood and involve discussion of highly technical concepts, including abnormal automaticity in the pulmonary vein areas of the left atrium and reentry. How far attendings want to go in discussing the current understanding of relevant disease mechanisms depends on their expertise and time constraints. Gathering a group of challenging cases to present to an invited colleague with "hands-on" experience is one way to make sure that these fundamental issues get discussed, even on very busy services. Finally, recall that even the most elegant of mechanistic explanations are likely to be incomplete and perhaps fundamentally incorrect. For example, our understandings of mechanisms of both MAT and atrial fibrillation continue to evolve, despite decades of study.

One of the most revolutionary examples of mechanistic reappraisals comes from gastroenterology. The pathophysiological link between the bacterium *Helicobacter pylori* and most peptic ulcers was not recognized until the 1980s, through the initially controversial work of two Australian physicians, Dr. Barry Marshall and Dr. Robin Warren. Their discovery, overturning decades of conventional wisdom and medical/surgical dogma about the noninfectious hydrochloric acid–related mechanism of ulcer disease was recognized with the 2005 Nobel Prize in Physiology or Medicine. Perhaps the commonly posed attending's round question "What is the underlying mechanism?" should be replaced with "What is our current understanding of the putative mechanisms, and what are the cutting-edge areas of debate and research?"

MINI-SUMMARY

- When confronting a clinical diagnostic problem, always ask the 3½ key questions:
- What is the Dx? What else could it be (DDx)? Dx and DDx should be considered as joint or tethered questions. In the DDx category, always leave an open category for something that you are not considering.
- What caused it (etiology)? Multiple factors may be at play.
- What to do about it (Rx/Tx)? Consider all the options.
- Remember that these practical questions are intended to enlarge consideration of alternative diagnoses and therapies, not to replace essential discussion of mechanisms of the relevant disease processes.

PART 2

MEDICAL MASTERIES

$E = MC^3$: *ERROR REDUCTION EQUALS MOTIVATION TIMES COMMUNICATION TO THE POWER OF 3*

Perhaps the history of the errors of mankind, all things considered, is more valuable and interesting than that of their discoveries.
—BENJAMIN FRANKLIN, 1706–1790

Victory has 100 fathers; defeat is an orphan.
—Quoted by President John F. Kennedy following the failed Bay of Pigs invasion of Cuba (1961). This is perhaps the most cited version of the original quote, attributed to Italian diplomat Count Caleazzo Ciano. But good quotes, like victories, often have multiple parents.

EXAMPLE: MINI-CASE REPORT

A 31-year-old man with pancytopenia was diagnosed with mast cell leukemia. The treatment plan centered on allogeneic stem cell transplantation. His care was transferred to a new team midway through his admission. Verbal and written sign-outs were given the day before the new house staff team came on service and his chart records were

---

Becoming a Consummate Clinician: What Every Student, House Officer, and Hospital Practitioner Needs to Know, First Edition.
Ary L. Goldberger and Zachary D. Goldberger.

reviewed by the new team. The electronic medical record reported NKDA (no known drug allergies).

Overnight, the cross-covering resident physician was notified that the patient had a temperature of 38.6°C and a heart rate of 110/min, but was normotensive. He was given acetaminophen 325 mg orally. One hour later, the patient's temperature had risen to 39.2°C, his heart rate to 120/min, but remained normotensive. A review of the medication list revealed that, despite an extensive antibiotic regimen, he was not being covered for methicillin-resistant *Staphylococcus aureus* (MRSA) infection. Vancomycin 1.0 g IV was administered. The patient was told he was being given "medicine for the fever."

Fifteen minutes after the infusion, he vomited and fell in the bathroom. His blood pressure was now 90/60 mmHg, heart rate 130/min, and he was tachypneic (25 breaths/min), with an SpO_2 of 85%. He was placed on a 100% oxygen via a nonrebreather face mask, treated empirically with a standard anaphylaxis protocol, and transferred to the ICU.

The following morning, a known allergy to vancomycin was "discovered," which had been documented previously in three places: the medical admission record, prior discharge summaries, and his allergy notification wristband.

At least five medical errors occurred here. We revisit this "index" case later. An important underlying theme of this book, and a major preoccupation of virtually all twenty-first-century medical endeavors, is how to reduce errors. The "equation" in the chapter title is not a miscue on the authors' part or a deconstruction of Einstein's mass–energy equivalence law. Instead, the heading is intended to convey a central message about the importance of communication and motivation in preventing and treating the epidemic of medical errors. In essence, all the chapters in the book deal with enhancing communication and critical thinking—skills that should have, as positive side effects, the early recognition and prevention of errors.

The cumulative cost in human health, lives, and monetary expenditures is staggering. Medication errors of the type described in the opening case are particularly frequent, but comprise only one component of a vast nosology of fumbles, stumbles, and lapses. Fortunately, the patient in that case did not die but could have, and his hospital stay was extended by several extra days in the ICU. In addition, he was given an antianaphylactic regimen that included high-dose corticosteroids, which themselves could have adversely affected his already compromised immune system.

Until recently, this topic was relatively unaddressed and under-researched, a part of the "dark matter of medicine": that is, something of enormous importance that is hidden from view. The subject of medical errors, discussed here from the particular perspective of trainees and hospital-based clinicians, has appropriately become a major topic in the medical literature and the media. The deafening silence on the importance of medical errors in this country was quietly broken with the publication of the landmark November 1999 monograph entitled *To Err Is Human: Building a Safer Healthcare System*, published by the Institute of Medicine. Although the topic of medical errors had been written about before, this publication issued a shot heard round the medical world. The opening sentences combine the quiet urgency and stark factuality akin to an Edward R. Murrow documentary:

> Health care in the United States is not as safe as it should be—and can be. At least 44,000 people, and perhaps as many as 98,000 people, die in hospitals each year as a result of medical errors that could have been prevented, according to estimates from two major studies. Even using the lower estimate, preventable medical errors in hospitals exceed attributable deaths to such feared threats as motor-vehicle wrecks, breast cancer, and AIDS.*

Yet, over a decade later, the problem of medical errors continues to be a national epidemic. The scope, costs, and persistence of the problem, coupled with the seeming intractability of "curing" multiple

---

*Of note, Rodney Hayward and Tim Hofer, in a 2001 *JAMA* article, reexamined these statistics, and found a great deal of interrater reliability when expert reviewers were asked to review charts for errors. In addition, the issue of whether these purported errors had implications for patient care was called into question.

classes of errors that seem eminently curable, indicate that current efforts are clearly insufficient. In an era where networking and communication capabilities are faster and more efficient than ever, how can these problems still be so prevalent?

This question is widely discussed and debated. Indeed, one might turn the question cephalad—on its head—and assert that modern medical practice is actually the perfect cauldron for augmenting, not minimizing, the likelihood of errors: Medicine is more complicated than in previous eras. More drugs are available, including those with highly potent effects that can disable clotting and immune systems as part of their therapeutic effects. Polypharmacy creates multidrug interactions for which no satisfactory models or mechanisms yet exist.

Our patients take a raft of supplemental therapies which may not be inquired about or reported but which can have profound interactions with "approved" medications. For example, use of garlic supplements may decrease the plasma concentrations of saquinavir and possibly other protease inhibitors used to treat HIV/AIDS. (The mechanism is not known but may involve induction of CYP450 metabolism or alterations of P-glycoprotein transport.) We rely on

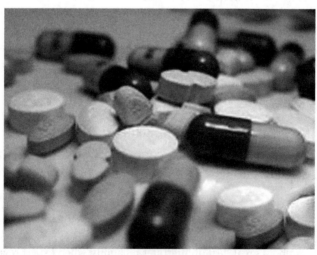

The polypharmacy approach can *create* a variety of problems as it *solves* others.

technologies that are more daunting and more remote from the bedside, making us depend almost entirely on the expertise of colleagues with whom we may never communicate directly and interactively. The reality is that it takes far less time to read a radiology report than to talk with the radiologists reading your patient's PET (positron emission tomographic) scan or to review it in person with them. Patient "throughput" is faster.

Patients may request or demand therapies (e.g., antibiotics for viral upper respiratory infections) that are not indicated and can lead to drug reactions and antibiotic resistance. Our fractured health care system deemphasizes prevention and transforms the avoidable or more readily treatable conditions into urgent ones or emergencies (e.g., poor dental care breeds abscesses; obesity promotes diabetes and its myriad of complications). Patients coming in for surgery are often older and have multiple comorbidities (i.e., they are more infirm). Specialties and subspecialties have become more focused to accommodate increased therapeutic options and an explosive knowledge base, but human physiology stubbornly resists modularization and compartmentalization.

These and other factors, while giving plausible explanations for the high prior probability of errors, do not account for their seeming intractability. Shouldn't some of the same factors that make errors more likely (more advanced technology and increased knowledge) help decrease errors by enhancing communication and expertise? We know more and can disseminate that information faster. So what is so wrong?

In our opinion, the seemingly "treatment-resistant" problem of medical errors relates in a very important way to the fact that this part of medicine is still something of an outlier, a topic brought up in selected conferences but not yet granted sufficient academic status as one of the marquee features of medical education. We propose that this topic should not only be part of the interstitial curriculum, the focus of this book. *Instead, all medical and nursing schools, house staff programs, and hospitals should consider the syndrome of medical errors as a central component of their core curricula, beginning in orientation and continuing throughout training and postgraduate education.*

DEFINING MEDICAL ERRORS: DO WE KNOW THEM WHEN WE SEE THEM?

We have used the term *medical error* without defining it formally. In a sense, by using an undefined term, we have ourselves committed a type of scientific error that speaks to a simultaneous lapse of rigor and communication. However, this semantic failing is unlikely to be listed in any medical error checklist.

The first steps toward curing errors would seem to be recognizing and acknowledging them (see Exhibit 7.1). But even more basically, it is important to ask "What is your definition of a medical error?" Or do you consider it one of those difficult terms that we all seem to know the meaning of but which generate different written definitions? Perhaps the most famous example of this paradoxical disconnect between the obvious and the definable is immortalized in former U.S. Supreme Court Justice Potter Stewart's oft-cited (non)-definition of obscenity: "I know it when I see it. . . ." Accordingly, do you have additions to Exhibit 7.1?

Clearly, the case presented earlier is an unequivocal example of a medical error. We all know it when we see or hear about a case like

EXHIBIT 7.1   Classification of Medical Errors

Diagnostic
    Error or delay in diagnosis
    Failure to employ tests indicated
    Use of outmoded tests or therapy
    Failure to act on results of monitoring or testing
Treatment-related
    Error in the performance of an operation, procedure, or test
    Error in administering the treatment
    Error in the dose or method of using a drug
    Avoidable delay in treatment or in responding to an abnormal test
    Inappropriate (not indicated) care
Prevention failures
    Failure to provide prophylactic treatment
    Inadequate monitoring or follow-up of treatment
Technical failures
    Equipment failure

Source: From Leape L. et al. Preventing medical injury. Qual Rev Bull. 1993;19:144–149. Reprinted with permission.

this where a patient is given a medication to which he or she is known to be allergic. Unfortunately, we hear about them all too often. The most egregious medical lapses become the topics of appropriately eye-grabbing feature stories:

> Dr. Lawrence K. Altman, writing in *The New York Times* on December 11, 2001, reported that at least 150 times since 1996 surgeons in hospitals in this country have operated on the wrong arm, leg, eye, kidney, or other body part, or even on the wrong patient. The figure does not include near misses—when surgeons started to operate on the wrong site or patient—because no one collects such information.

Puzzlingly, ridding the medical system of nightmare errors in which surgeries are performed on the wrong part of the body or even the wrong person still remains a challenge, as the newspaper story shown in Figure 7.1 indicates.

One would reasonably think that these types of errors should be fully preventable by widely touted "system" approaches that involve instituting multiple layers of surveillance and cross-checking. But somehow they continue to persist. Operations still occur on the wrong

Hasbro doctor begins operating on wrong part of child's mouth

01:00 AM EDT on Thursday, May 14, 2009

By Felice J. Freyer

Journal Medical Writer

A surgeon on Monday began operating on the wrong part of a child's mouth during surgery to correct a cleft palate at Hasbro Children's Hospital, the fifth wrong-site surgery in Rhode Island since 2007.

The error was noticed during surgery and the correct procedure then performed, "with good results," Dr. Timothy J. Babineau, president of Rhode Island Hospital, of which Hasbro is part., said in a statement. "The patient is in good condition and we do not anticipate any further complications related to this error," he said.

FIGURE 7.1   The importance of presurgical preparation. Reprinted with permission from *Providence Journal Bulletin.*

side, drug dosages are confused, and biopsies get assigned to the wrong patients. How is that possible?

So What Is a Medical Error?

The definition of medical errors is not without controversy. Current definitions usually emphasize preventable aspects of medical practice that actually harm or have the potential to cause harm to a patient. Following is a definition of medication errors proposed by the National Coordinating Council for Medication Error Reporting and Prevention that could be generalized to include many other types of medical mistakes.

> A medication error is any preventable event that may cause or lead to inappropriate medication use or patient harm while the medication is in the control of the health care professional, patient, or consumer. Such events may be related to professional practice, health care products, procedures, and systems, including prescribing; order communication; product labeling, packaging, and nomenclature; compounding; dispensing; distribution; administration; education; monitoring; and use.

Along with evolving consensus definitions, clinicians and others have been challenged with the task of deriving newer and more relevant classifications of what are sometimes mistakenly confused with *iatrogenic diseases*. Keep in mind that medical errors are not the same as complications or as traditional iatrogenic (treatment-caused) pathologies. A key component of medical errors has to do with their preventability. Some complications—for example, stroke after aortic valve surgery in an 85-year-old man—may not be easily preventable. They often come "bundled" with the procedure. Corticosteroid-induced diabetes mellitus in a patient with lupus erythematosus is iatrogenic, but may be unavoidable.

Returning to the Definition

The National Council's definition of a medical error is broad and, if read literally, contains quite controversial, almost radical language. If you are an attending, try it out on your colleagues and trainees during rounds. According to this definition, aspects of the direct advertisement of drugs to consumers by the pharmaceutical industry might fall under its penumbra.

Less controversially, the example at the beginning of this chapter is clearly an extreme demonstration of a medication error and constitutes one of the most preventable causes of medication-related morbidity and even mortality—a patient is given a medication to which he is known (and documented by wristband) to be allergic. This is the prototype of a procedural, and one would hypothesize readily fixable, class of errors. Another example would be administration of a drug with a sound-alike name instead of the one that is actually intended. An extensive list of look- and sound-alike drug names that have led to confusion is published by the Institute for Safe Medicine Practices. This list includes both generic and brand names. For example, dispensing Adderal (a central nervous systemic stimulant composed of amphetamine-type compounds) instead of Inderal (a nonselective beta 1 and beta 2 receptor blocking agent) could lead to disastrous cardiovascular effects (tachycardia, increased contractility, and hypertension) in the most vulnerable patients: those with preexisting coronary artery disease or tachyarrhythmias.

Other medication errors are far more subtle, involving, for example, addition of one drug that alters the metabolism of another that the patient is already taking. This type of "double-whammy" drug interaction was discussed earlier for a patient taking amiodarone and digitalis. The prevention of potentially deleterious drug interactions requires a fundamentally different, higher order of information, knowledge of pharmacology, not just allergy cross checks and medication nomenclature. The problem of drug interactions is exacerbated further by the difficulties in identifying which drugs a patient has recently or is currently taking (called medication reconciliation, discussed in Chapter 1), adherence, confounding effects of age (e.g., decreased renal function with aging), gender and other genetic factors, and the fact that polypharmacy may induce interactions that have not even been described.

Such errors should be fully preventable by system approaches that involve instituting multiple layers of surveillance and cross-checking. But somehow they are not, or at least not yet, preventable. Operations still occur on the wrong side, drug dosages are confused, and biopsies get assigned to the wrong patients.

But the most difficult medical mistakes to correct, and ultimately prevent, are those that are not readily detected and sometimes never even recognized: *cognitive errors.* Cognitive failures are much more difficult to classify and cannot be cured by implementing an aviation-type checklist. One class of cognitive lapses includes failures to look at data creatively and imaginatively and to re-look at data to catch hidden but accessible information critical to a patient's well-being. Avoiding such cognitive errors is a multifaceted endeavor that exercises all of our training. Fortunately, addressing a number of specific and recurrent themes may improve our level of clinical care and confidence. These skills are readily within the grasp of all students of medicine. For example, you can train yourself to:

- Frame differential diagnoses in the most effective ways (Chapter 6)
- Ask the questions that are you *not* asking—unaddressed questions that may have lethal consequences if ignored (Chapter 1)
- Think about clues to missing or mistaken diagnoses that may be contained in outlier values (Chapter 11)

THE FLIP SIDE

We all agree that giving medications to which patients are allergic, giving an incorrect medication (Zyprexa instead of Zyrtec), or giving an incorrect dosage are clear examples of medical errors. But it is also useful to ask: What is left out of the National Council's definition of medication-related errors above? The answers might include failure to give drugs for appropriate indications and giving the right drugs (e.g., antibiotics for pneumonia), but definitive therapy is not initiated until hours later by the ward team.

Other errors stem from a failure to exercise common standards of practice, such as hand-washing before and after patient contact. The work of Ignaz Semmelweis is responsible for the practice of frequent hand-washing in the hospital. Semmelweis practiced at a maternity hospital in Vienna in the mid-nineteenth century. In one of the two maternity wards, a disproportionate number of women were dying of puerperal fever, often referred to as "childbed fever." The breakthrough occurred when he learned that a friend and colleague, Jakob Kolletschka, a forensic pathologist, died following an autopsy in which he was accidentally poked with a student's scalpel. Kolletschka's postmortem exam revealed that the cause of his death was puerperal fever. Semmelweis hypothesized that "particles" present on the hands were causing the infection introduced during the obstetric physical examination. This theory also accounted for the fact that the patients of midwives in the other maternity ward, who did not perform autopsies, had a much lower mortality rate.

Only two decades after he died were his "evidence-based" findings generally accepted. By then, the germ theory of disease, proposed by Louis Pasteur and Joseph Lister, offered hard evidence to support Semmelweis's empirical observations. Further detail of this remarkable and brave discovery can be read in Semmelweis's autobiography, *Etiology, Concept and Prophylaxis of Childbed Fever*. It should not escape notice that getting physicians to wash their hands before and after every patient encounter remains a contemporary challenge on many hospital wards.

ERRORS THAT FLY BELOW THE RADAR

An underdiscussed category of medical errors, relevant to medications as well as other therapeutically motivated interventions are those that currently have no classification schema. These errors literally fly below the radar and only when they cross a critical threshold, sometimes with critical side effects, do they get noticed; or they may not be classified as errors at all. One major, potentially unclassified error is calling a code on a patient whose status is "do not resuscitate" (see Chapter 4 for an illustrative case history). A more subtle version of this mistake is not to define clearly the code status of patients or to fail to update it and notify other members of the team when one of their patients' code statuses has changed. We mention a few other examples here and then challenge our readers to come up with actual and potential errors that may escape identification and classification.

The "One Size (or a Few) Fits All" Syndrome

Medications are typically prescribed in fixed, discrete dosages because of the way that the pills (or capsules, etc.) are manufactured. This reality greatly restricts a clinician's flexibility in prescribing "intermediate" or very low amounts of a medication. This limitation is particularly relevant in prescribing for very elderly patients and for small patients. The lowest usual dosage of some medication for the "average adult" may actually be quite high for a 95-lb 90-year-old woman. For antihypertensive medications, those affecting sinus and AV node function (e.g., beta-blockers and calcium-channel blockers) and those affecting mental function, even modest "overtreatment" imposed by the lowest available dosage may be especially impactful.

The reflex of clinicians to "reach for" a fixed dose of some medication is motivated by convenience and reinforced by evidence-based data (e.g., double-blind randomized controlled trials), which tend to employ such regimens. For example, in the Heart Outcomes Prevention Evaluation (HOPE) trial, a single dose (10 mg) of the angiotensin-converting enzyme inhibitor ramipril was compared with placebo or vitamin E in subjects who were not known to have a reduced left ventricular ejection fraction to assess effects on cardiac outcomes: namely, death, myocardial infarction, and stroke (N Engl J Med. 2000;342:145–153).

Errors That Harm Doctors

Physical harm to doctors due to medical practice has received considerable attention (e.g., needle sticks that carry a risk of HIV or hepatitis infections). But doctors can also be harmed psychologically by the harm that they inadvertently cause to patients. We can become collateral damage in our own campaigns against disease. The hidden costs to the system in terms of physician burnout, guilt, and even depression and suicide are substantial.

Adverse effects of medical errors on caregivers are highlighted in a 2007 *New England Journal of Medicine* Perspective article by Dr. Tom Delbanco and Dr. Sigall Bell entitled "Guilty, Afraid, and Alone—Struggling with Medical Error." The authors point out that medical error may evoke profound feelings of guilt not only in family members but also in the physicians and other team members caring for the patient. "Clinicians who feel guilty after a medical error may have parallel feelings of fear—fear for their reputation, their job, their license, and their own future as well as that of their patient." Fatal mistakes may disable caregivers.

BACK TO THE INDEX CASE

What went wrong in the case presented to begin this discussion? The short answer is: pretty much everything. A summary list that might make its way to a quality assurance board would include:

- Incomplete or inaccurate house staff sign-outs
- Information not immediately accessible during a busy night shift
- Pharmacy-dispensed medication without double-checking the medical record
- Nursing or medical staff did not identify and report an allergy bracelet and update the chart
- Incomplete communication of treatment plan with patient

The fact that all these lapses occurred in sequence or in parallel is a more *global* lapse that makes this case notable but not unique. A common theme of these individual failures is flawed communication:

doctor to doctor, nurse to nurse, nurse to doctor, pharmacy to clinicians, and clinicians with the patient. We leave it as an exercise for trainees and attendings alike to come up with cures for this type of problem. What we want to conclude with as part of this challenge is a rarely emphasized but essential facet of the prevention and correction of medical errors: the role of attending rounds.

ROUNDING UP ERRORS

The importance of *motivation* in reducing medical errors was emphasized in the $E = mc^3$ formulation. Almost every case you will participate in has some feature that is not optimal. This assertion is not a statement of universal liability but of human (im)perfectability. A key attribute of clinicians in training and those in practice is not to be perfect but to learn from our mistakes and the miscues of others and then to generalize that learning, to the extent possible, throughout the system. The prevention of mistakes requires the inculcation of what Dr. Mark Seidel, Beth Israel Deaconess Medical Center, and other health care leaders, have termed a permeative "culture of quality."

Medical errors (such as the military–political defeats in the opening JFK quote) have many sources ("fathers") and often relate to lapses in information acquisition and transmission. Some of the most notorious and seemingly "curable" of these errors have motivated the development of supposedly fail-safe methods to ensure that surgeons operate on the correct (not necessarily the "right") side; that drug dosages are appropriate for age, weight, and renal and hepatic function; that blood transfusions are administered correctly; and that potentially dangerous drug interactions are identified ahead of time and averted.

Such errors have become classified as "system" errors because they often indicate a breakdown in the network of surveillance and protection measures designed to maximize patient safety. Like other human disasters, their occurrence often leads to uncovering multiple lapses in the "system," involving physicians, nurses, and pharmacists, as in the drug error presented here. Their reoccurrence and its prevention arguably pose two of the most pressing challenges to clinical medicine in this century.

Therefore, we suggest that an essential feature of virtually all case presentations be some discussion of "room for improvement" and where relevant, of the identification of actual mistakes or near misses that may serve as the basis of enhanced patient care. This component should not be viewed as less essential than the presentation of the vital signs. Errors, in their own way, *are* vital signs.

MINI-SUMMARY

- Preventable errors, despite their nearly universal acknowledgment, continue to be endemic, costing thousands of lives, with enormous economic and social costs to the system.
- Medical students, house staff trainees, and attendings should not consider rounds complete without discussion on each case of how some aspects of care could be enhanced, and a frank discussion of preventable medical errors when they occur.

CHAPTER 8

EVIDENCE-BASED MEDICINE: WHAT AND WHERE IS THE EVIDENCE?

Nor is there anything to be relied upon in Physick [clinical practice] but an exact knowledge of medicinal physiology (founded on observation, not principles), semiotics [signs], method of curing, and tried . . . medicines.

—JOHN LOCKE, 1823

. . . the code is more what you'd call "guidelines" than actual rules.
—Pirate Hector Barbossa in *Pirates of the Caribbean: The Curse of the Black Pearl*, Disney, 2003.

One of the most widely used terms in modern medicine is *evidence-based medicine* (EBM). Supportive evidence for this statement is provided by the over 70,000 citations retrievable under this three-word term in PubMed. The term has assumed almost mantra-like qualities. Clearly, all clinicians want and should always aim to practice compassionate medicine informed both by rigorous biostatistics and basic science: another way of saying *evidence-based practice*. The opening quote from British philosopher and dean of empiricism John Locke uncannily reads like a "back to the future" prescription. It should be

Becoming a Consummate Clinician: What Every Student, House Officer, and Hospital Practitioner Needs to Know, First Edition.
Ary L. Goldberger and Zachary D. Goldberger.
© 2012 Wiley-Blackwell. Published 2012 by John Wiley & Sons, Inc.

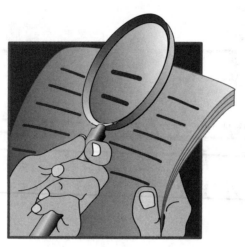

The evidence: What/where is it?

a clinical reflex to ask, especially before performing any therapeutic intervention: "What scientific knowledge base supports clinical decision making in this patient: using drugs, devices, or watching and waiting?" Alternatively phrased: "How good is the evidence, weighted by its reliability, for what we are proposing to do with my particular patient?"

In clinical practice, EBM has come to imply almost exclusively the use of some intervention, pharmacological or otherwise, that is supported by one (and preferably more) randomized controlled trials (RCTs), the statistical gold standard of clinical studies. Increasingly, the practice of EBM is becoming incorporated into sets of guidelines that are issued and updated by various specialty societies. Guidelines of this type also rate how strong the evidence is to support a given form of therapy.

The term *evidence-based medicine* was first used in print in a historic 1992 publication of the *Journal of the American Medical Association* (*JAMA*), by Dr. Gordon Guyatt and colleagues at the Ontario Ministry of Health, as part of a working group of biomedical experts from a variety of international institutions. The field of EBM was strongly rooted in the burgeoning science of clinical trials and a new wave of research that looked critically at various aspects of medical practice that previously had been taken for granted.

CLINICAL USE OF EBM

The application of EBM (especially via RCTs) has deconstructed a number of long-held medical practices that were useless or even dangerous, One example is the discrediting of the use of conventional hormone replacement therapy as a routine part of the management of peri- and postmenopausal women. Another is the repudiation of certain antiarrhythmic agents to prevent death after myocardial infarction.

On the constructive side, via careful RCTs, EBM has led to multiple lifesaving or prolonging advances, including the routine use of aspirin in the treatment of acute coronary syndromes and the use of beta-blockers in patients after myocardial infarction and, counterintuitively, in many patients with heart failure.

EBM is important for at least three reasons: (1) for supporting clinical decision making and consensus guidelines on what to do, (2) for indicating what "therapies" have been debunked and should be discontinued in their current implementation because reliable studies show that these practices have no effect or have proven toxicities, and (3) for identifying gray zones where data are insufficient to make firm recommendations so that additional studies and analysis are indicated.

From a student's point of view, discussions of EBM are essential. But there are a number of aspects of EBM that receive limited attention on the ward and in some textbook discussions. Next we provide a brief overview of some of these considerations.

Busy clinicians make hundreds of decisions a day. These decisions fall into two general classes: those that that are explicit and those that are implicit. For example, the decision to use an antibiotic for therapy of abdominal wall cellulitis—the choice of a particular compound, its preparation, the route of administration (oral or parenteral), the overall daily dosage, the dosing interval, and the duration of therapy—are explicit decisions. However, others, such as the decision as to whether and how to pursue underlying immunologic deficiencies, are implicit.

Although RCTs are a gold standard, their applicability to the patient you are treating ($n = 1$) is always open to question. For example, if you are using as evidence the findings of a given trial or, even better, a series of trials, it is important to review the literature. Keep in mind that as useful as RCTs are, they always have exclusion criteria, and even among patients who qualify, only a small percentage actually get accepted.

As a clinician, you are essentially almost always treating all-comers, as there are no selection biases or exclusions in most major medical centers. In contrast, randomized trials are necessarily "over-selected"; that is, they have exclusion criteria for patients who want to participate. They also do not include patients who are eligible and qualify (the "healthy volunteer effect") but choose not to participate (e.g., patients who don't respond to radio or other advertisements; patients who are interviewed and accepted but then recuse themselves) or patients who are disqualified based on regional, geographic, or other considerations. Efforts to include a diverse patient population—a major preoccupation of the NIH, human subjects committees, pharmaceutical manufacturers, and biostatisticians for different reasons—are only partially successful in coping with such challenges.

THE NEED TO LOOK AT DATA CRITICALLY

As a student or house officer you should always go back to the original studies used to support a particular form of therapy in your patients. Next, ask whether in fact the patient you are caring for would have even qualified for entry into the study in the first place. Or question whether or not the patient would have been excluded by age (too young or too old), comorbid conditions (e.g., alcoholism or dementia, hepatobiliary or renal disease), certain medications, and so on. And consider how these disqualifying categories were assessed (e.g., for renal disease by serum creatinine or estimated creatinine clearance?). Conversely, if at first glance your patient fits into all the inclusionary "bins," you should ask two other questions: How well does your own patient actually qualify? How feasible is it to follow the study protocol in your practice?

As an example, suppose that your patient is a 78-year-old woman and that the age criterion for the available evidence-based (randomized control) studies is 21 to 80 years. Your patient seems to be accommodated by this range. But perhaps in actuality only 10 patients out of 1500 studied were actually in the very elderly (75 to 80 years old) category and most were men. In such cases it would be helpful to have access to additional data (e.g., well-obtained observational reports) that are reassuring about the use of the specific therapy in elderly women. These data may or may not be available, or to the extent they have been acquired they may not be accessible.

Another potential problem with applying studies based on large numbers of carefully selected individuals to the $n = 1$ patient under your care is illustrated by the following example. Implantable cardioverter-defibrillator (ICD) therapy for primary prevention of sudden cardiac arrest or death in patients with substantial heart muscle dysfunction after myocardial infarction is now a standard of care. To quote from the 2008 ACC/AHA/HRS guidelines: "ICD therapy is indicated in patients with LVEF [left ventricular ejection fraction] less than or equal to 35% due to prior myocardial infarction who are at least 40 days postmyocardial infarction and are in NYHA functional class II or III." This is considered as a strongly advised (class I) recommendation with substantial evidence (level A) to support it. The reliability of the supportive evidence has been reviewed elsewhere. For our purposes, imagine that you are a clinician taking care of a patient 6 months after an MI who is found by echocardiogram to have an LVEF estimated to be 40%. According to the guidelines, this patient would not qualify for an ICD. However, echocardiographic estimates of LVEF carry (almost always) unstated error (±) bars which may well be ±5%. So, does the patient now qualify since her LVEF is within one or two standard deviations of the mean? Or suppose you obtain a nuclear scan which gives the LVEF as 34%. Do you choose the lower or the higher estimate of ventricular function as the basis of recommending a preventive therapy that carries its own side effects (especially the chance of unnecessary and painful shocks due to misfiring of the device)? What are the error bars of this measure? What does the evidence tell you to do, and what is the evidenced-based way of resolving such uncertainties that pervade medicine?

Attempting to incorporate the results of recent evidence into your own clinical practice is commendable, after appreciating the appropriate exclusions of RCTs. However, remember that RCTs epitomize the highest form of clinical efficacy, which, in itself, is different from clinical effectiveness. *Efficacy* refers to how the therapy being studied *should* work, but most often in the context of ideal settings. Initial studies usually are based on a carefully selected group of patients (many, as above, who are not like the ones to whom you are attempting to apply the evidence), who are carefully followed up by the trial administrators and found to be nearly 100% compliant with their medication and follow-up visits/lab tests. Clinical effectiveness, in contrast, speaks to the effect in real-world practice.

A NEW PARADIGM?

The 1992 paper describing the original intent of the EBM working group should be read and reread by those who profess to practice its tenets. The document is more nuanced and less dogmatic than current discussions might suggest. In defining what they labeled as a "new paradigm," the authors suggested three guiding assumptions or propositions (as quoted in their own words):

1. Clinical experience and the development of clinical instincts are a crucial and necessary part of becoming a competent physician. Many aspects of clinical practice cannot, or will not, ever be adequately tested.
2. The study and understanding of basic mechanisms of disease are necessary but insufficient guides for clinical practice.
3. Understanding certain rules of evidence is necessary to correctly interpret literature on causation, prognosis, diagnostic tests, and treatment strategy.

What is the evidence that EBM is actually a new paradigm? Certainly not the first proposition noted above. The primacy of experience and clinical instincts (judgment) is universally recognized as a key to practice. The second statement only acknowledges the obvious—that our understanding of basic mechanisms is always incomplete and often incorrect with respect to important aspects. Even full knowledge of basic mechanisms (which is never available) does not translate into successful and definitive therapeutic efforts, although more knowledge is always helpful. The third assumption is also hardly radical but rather a call, or even an alarm, for more critical thinking about the nature of data supporting a given intervention or approach.

What made the conceptual framework of EBM plausibly a new paradigm is the combination of all three central components: an *emergent* property that is not contained in any one of them. Indeed, read separately they sound rather like business as usual. But when you activate the cognitive machine of EBM by flipping on all three switches, you get an unexpected result. You deconstruct authority. You pull the rug out from under the conventional wisdom and from top-down authority, whose only justification for a given line of approach is often tradition. "We do it this way because we have always done it this way."

EBM is democratizing and distributive of knowledge. It encourages and even requires discussion and dissent. You should assume that all forms of prognostic, diagnostic, and therapeutic activity are flawed until otherwise demonstrated. Just because an attending says so doesn't make it true. However, EBM also deconstructs itself. The same rigor it requires of other past approaches must be applied to those that sail under the flag of EBM. Just because an RCT provides some evidence to favor one approach over others does not mean that the study is the last word on the subject. In addition, EBM is not an abdication of practice to biostatisticians and others who do not work on basic mechanisms or who have not had years of clinical and observational experience treating real patients.

The sublime subversiveness of EBM is that it always forces us to ask, "Why do we do it this way?" Yet it does not disrespect the notion that the continuity of clinical judgment plays a major role, especially if years of experience suggest that one or another approach is a good one and if no credible study has addressed the problem rigorously or definitively. Most of all, it does not undercut the essential importance of understanding basic mechanisms of disease. Rather, it invites a high level of skepticism about explanations parading as mechanistic insights. Just because a study has been published in a high-impact peer-reviewed journal does not make it correct or reproducible. Further, as discussed in Chapter 9, many adverse off-target effects of drugs only become apparent years after a drug has been approved by the U.S. Food and Drug Administration and released for general clinical use.

LIMITATIONS OF RCTs

Most of the questions posed in medical practice will never be resolved by RCTs, for reasons of cost, feasibility, or ethics. For example, an RCT will not be undertaken when the evidence of efficacy or effectiveness is considered too overwhelming to test. An example is surgical intervention vs. medical therapy with antibiotics for acute appendicitis. However, RCTs might usefully examine different modes of surgical approach (e.g., laparoscopic vs. conventional).

One inherent limitation of large RCTs (i.e., those trials with the most statistical power) is the reality that medicine is like a high-speed train. Often by the time a study has ended (or even begun enrolling patients) new modalities are available (e.g., use of the first generation of cardiac stents was followed by the introduction of those with different types of coating, especially drug-eluting varieties). For technology-based studies, new versions or embodiments of the original intervention are likely to come at increasingly shorter intervals, making it difficult or impossible to play catch-up.

Another limitation is that RCTs necessarily make a trade-off between statistical rigor and flexibility. This conflict applies to studies of drugs or devices. Thus, only a limited number of drug dosages might be tested in a given study, and differences in the modality of giving a drug (e.g., time of day; single vs. multiple doses) may not be tested at all.

A more controversial source of bias in RCTs is that they often compare a specific branded drug with placebo. Unsponsored or "orphan" compounds are less likely to be studied, especially when support comes from industry.

One of the purported strengths of RCTs is that they often include large numbers of subjects, conferring statistical power. Paradoxically, the "large n" value is also a source of inherent weakness, especially when it comes to applying the findings to the $n = 1$ setting, where you are treating one patient whose pathophysiology, social context, and multiple unmeasured variables almost certainly make the person quite different from the "average patient" reported in a given study. Indeed, the notion of an "average patient" is both a medical and a statistical fiction. Students and trainees need to learn how to assess RCTs for hidden as well as overt biases and how to avoid the pitfall of what Drs. David Kent and Rodney Hayward describe in their 2007 article on the "Limitations of Applying Summary Results of Clinical Trials to Individual Patients," published in *JAMA*.

Another limitation of reporting RCTs and most other clinical trials is that the actual data points that underlie the statistical analyses are rarely, if ever, published. Instead, readers are presented with data summarized as mean±variance-based values and, sometimes, ranges and confidence intervals. The data may be represented by bar graphs or fancier "whisker plots." But what is "missing in action" (e.g., not usually even made available as a supplement or available by request) are the individual data points that were used to make these plots and do the analyses.

Without such *open-access* data (of course, protecting patient confidentiality), the published study has insurmountable limitations. Imagine if reports of genomic or proteomic findings did not present the actual sequences—they wouldn't be publishable. *Yet RCTs are published routinely without showing any of the fundamental data.* The unavailability of primary data greatly limits reanalysis and data mining. This culture of sequestration of the original data also creates a closed-access bias; students and clinicians routinely assume that the summary statistics given in peer-reviewed studies are the basic data—they are not.

Readers should be cognizant of these important tensions and the active controversies in contemporary medicine between advocates of EBM who cite the robustness of findings based on large numbers of patients and those who caution against overgeneralizing from large n to the $n = 1$ you are seeing in the clinic or ward. For example, the term *aggregate bias* has been suggested to characterize physicians who believe that large data sets used to develop clinical practice guidelines do not apply to individual patients (especially their own). However, this type of bias (often called ecological) may cut both ways if the aggregate data do not, in fact, include a sufficient number of patients matching key attributes of the patient they are seeing or, more subtly, if the mismatch is due to hidden variables that are not assessable based on the published data.

EVIDENCE-BASED MEDICINE AND MEDICAL SCIENCE: FINAL CAVEATS

As a final note, medical trainees in particular need to be aware of and guard against a subtle adverse effect of most discussion on rounds centering on EBM. The hazard is that empirical, nonfoundational science may be privileged over deeper understanding of the underlying pathophysiology, and the latter may even be ignored completely in such discussions. For example, the importance of beta-blockers in a wide range of patients with heart failure is now supported by multiple trials. However, students need to be aware of the pathophysiology of heart failure and the role of neurohumoral activation that probably underlies the success of this modality of therapy, despite its inherently negative inotropic effects. Preceptors conducting discussions of evidence-based interventions may be surprised when they ask students and house staff conversant with the clinical findings to discuss the mechanisms purportedly involved, what the drugs are actually doing, and what the side effects and toxicities of these interventions are.

Getting More Comfortable with the Certainty of Uncertainty in Medicine

One of the attractive, almost seductive features of EBM is that it seems to reduce the uncertainty the makes clinical decision making so difficult. However, as we have seen when the tools of EBM are turned on EBM itself, uncertainty is rarely quenched, and indeed is often increased.

From a more general perspective, students and trainees need to be explicitly aware that uncertainty is a universal attribute of human knowledge. In physics, the uncertainty principle is foundational to quantum mechanics (the microworld) and relates to the nonintuitive fact that the position and momentum of atomic and subatomic particles cannot be determined simultaneously with exact precision. Perhaps you fled physics not just because the math was unfathomable but because this type of uncertainty was intolerable. If so, medicine would be an ironic career choice. The reason is that uncertainties, albeit of a different type than those in the submicroscopic world, fully permeate the macroworld of medicine. Diagnoses are typically uncertain (for example, "Is my patient's dyspnea solely due to recurrent pulmonary emboli?"). Underscoring the importance of differential diagnoses ("What else could it be?"), you may uncover multiple contributory causes to the dyspnea (e.g., pulmonary emboli, heart failure, and obstructive lung disease).

Ockham's (Occam's) razor principle is named after fourteenth-century English friar, William of Ockham, who advised: Try to explain findings using the fewest assumptions. Also called the *principle of parsimony*, the edict is invoked by clinicians seeking an elegant, unifying cause or mechanism to account for a bunch of disparate, seemingly unrelated findings. When it works (e.g., a patient with polyneuropathy, fever, and AV heart block, all explained by Lyme disease), everyone cheers. But keep in mind the counterbalancing and cautionary notion, sometimes referred to as *Hickam's principle*: Patients can have as many diseases as they "damn well please." (See also Chapter 10.)

Furthermore, even where the diagnosis is apparently unambiguous (confirmed deep venous thrombosis and pulmonary emboli), the optimal management (what are the anticoagulant options, and which should we choose?) and the prognosis (what happens next?) can never be guaranteed or forecast precisely for an individual patient. Doctors almost always make decisions with incomplete information. But the "certainty of uncertainty," in addition to fostering humility and caution, also puts a premium on rigor of analysis and clarity of presentation. Paradoxically, the best strategies to handle clinical uncertainty involve managing some control over the information available, recognizing where the factual margins blur and the ambiguities reside; being able to communicate this information to colleagues as precisely and concisely as possible; and explaining it in nontechnical and nonalarming terms to patients.

When you present information in an unclear way, the complexities and ambiguities of the clinical data are magnified while simultaneously becoming more blurred. This double whammy is a bad combination in microscopy and medicine. The analogy to incoherent verbal presentations of complex cases would be to write out your history, physical, and other notes in an unreadable scrawl, a caricature of the "doctor's penmanship" syndrome. Cognitive and verbal illegibility are no less consequential than the oft-noted indecipherability of physician penmanship. (Computer-typed notes are increasingly obviating the latter problem, but with the side effects of fractured spelling and syntax. The added perils of cut-and-paste notes are discussed in Chapter 4.)

Quantitative vs. Pseudoquantitative Medicine

With these considerations in mind, students also need to be particularly mindful of hard numbers and other data tossed around during rounds that are masquerading as statistically-based, major-league knowledge. For example (you can fill in the blanks from something you may have heard on today's rounds): "X% of patients taking a given drug develop some serious side effect or complication" or "The sensitivity of a given test for some condition is Y%." These kinds of "evidence-based" data carry the semblance of certainty and solidity, but usually vaporize under more rigorous scrutiny.

As discussed previously, all clinical numbers come with uncertainty (error bars and a range), so a single value is almost never an adequate summary. These numbers typically derive from studies, or sometimes even a single report, of varying reliability and inevitable selection bias. It is very unusual on rounds to hear an attending say, for example: "The sensitivity of near-maximal exercise tests to detect myocardial ischemia in men presenting with chest discomfort of uncertain origin averages $X\%$ with a range of Y to $Z\%$ based on multiple studies." Students need to "get under the hood" of the numbers they read about or hear cited regarding their patients. What is the source of a resident's or attending's claim that the success rate for inducing remission in a given type of lymphoma with a certain regimen is $X\%$? Would our patient have been included in that trial, or would she have been excluded because of age, comorbidities, or other factors? Does the study report explicitly describe the outcome for someone in your patient's age group with comparable extent of disease? Do you and your colleagues know the estimated sensitivity and specificity of a test before the patient is sent for that exam, and what is your estimate of the pretest probability?

> As a working rule: Always assume that the statistics you are quoted are provisional if not frankly incorrect until you can validate them from a primary source. Even then, the numbers still may not be right!

EVIDENCE-BASED MEDICINE: CLINICAL INERTIA AND EXIT BLOCK SYNDROMES

This chapter has focused primarily on some of the weaknesses and limitations of contemporary EBM. In this concluding section, we want to note that sometimes clinical practice lags behind strong evidence or appears to ignore it entirely. Failure of caregivers to observe universal hand-washing procedures is one example. Others are more subtle. The term *clinical inertia* has been used to describe to the failure of physicians to initiate or intensify therapy when indicated by strong evidence (e.g., use of aspirin after myocardial infarction for secondary prevention). Perhaps this concept of inertia should be defined more widely to include sluggishness or resistance to changing a variety of clinical behaviors despite strong evidence for this change.

An example is the failure of many clinical laboratories and standard texts to adopt appropriate lower therapeutic ranges for the drug digoxin. Current data clearly support reducing the recommended therapeutic trough digoxin level range from the original, and still widely used, 0.8 to 2.0 ng/mL to much lower values (e.g., 0.5 to

0.8 ng/mL), both in the treatment of heart failure with systolic dys-function and in ventricular rate control with atrial fibrillation or flutter. Yet, although some influential resources have adapted these narrower ranges, others have failed to do so, including, at the time of this writing, some of the most widely read medical textbooks. Fur-thermore, even within some multiauthored texts, disparate recom-mendations are given in different chapters. In light of its low therapeutic margin of safety, the lack of evidence that the drug improves mortality (but overdose may be lethal) and the clinical instability of many of the patients to whom it is prescribed, the failure to universally adopt the lower therapeutic ranges recommended by cardiology specialty societies is surprising. The mechanisms for this example of evidence-based "exit block" are probably multiple and worthy of further study. In the meantime, trainees and attendings should be aware of this misalignment between well-documented evi-dence and laboratory guidelines for digoxin use. Whether other drug or metabolic levels also need to be critically reexamined and redefined is an open question invited by the case of digoxin.

MINI-SUMMARY

- The tools of evidence-based medicine or EBM (a posture of scientific skepticism, critical analysis, and constant reap-praisal) should always be used in evaluating any study or report claimed as "hard" evidence for a given diagnostic or therapeutic approach.
- Trying to "hoist the evidence on its own petard" is a fundamen-tal obligation of clinical science.
- Be on the lookout for clinical inertia and evidence-based exit block where clinical practice has failed to become fully aligned with strong evidence supporting a change in diagnosis or therapy.

CHAPTER 9

CAUTION! DANGEROUS BIOMEDICAL SEMANTICS AT WORK

> We don't see things as they are; we see things as we are.
> —Anaïs Nin (1903–1977), Cuban–French author and diarist

Senior as well as more junior clinicians are often victims of a hidden type of bias, one that we have created with our own biomedical terminology. This bias is camouflaged in the very words we use for drugs, biochemicals, and interventions. These terms are not deliberately intended to mislead, but unfortunately, that is often their consequence, sometimes with dangerous side effects.

SEMANTIC BIAS AND THE DRUGS YOU PRESCRIBE

Almost no attention is paid on the wards to *semantic sources of bias* that can warp your reading of the literature and create false expectations, as well as detour opportunities for scientific discovery. Most of these terms are indelibly inscribed in the language of medicine (and some are brand names). You need to be on the lookout for these medical "name games" and to compensate for them. Some may surprise you.

Becoming a Consummate Clinician: What Every Student, House Officer, and Hospital Practitioner Needs to Know, First Edition.
Ary L. Goldberger and Zachary D. Goldberger.
© 2012 Wiley-Blackwell. Published 2012 by John Wiley & Sons, Inc.

TABLE 9.1   Commonly Used Schema to Classify Cardiac Antiarrhythmic Drugs[a]

Class	Description
I	Sodium-channel blockers
IA	Depress phase 0 of action potential; delay conduction; prolong repolarization (phase III–IV); quinidine, procainamide, disopyramide
IB	Little effect on phase 0 of action potential in normal tissues; depress phase 0 in abnormal tissues; shorten repolarization or little effect; lidocaine, tocainide, mexiletine, dephenylhydantion
IC	Depress phase 0 of the action potential; markedly slow conduction in normal tissues; flecainide, propafenone
II	Beta-adrenergic blocking agents; acebutolol, atenolol, bisoprolol, carvedilol, metoprolol, nadolol, pindolol, propranolol, and others
III	Prolong action potential duration by increasing repolarization and refractoriness; amiodarone, dronedarone, sotalol, dofetilide, ibutilide
IV	Calcium-channel blockers; diltiazem, verapamil
Others	Digoxin, adenosine

[a]Drugs in classes IA and III may prolong the QT interval, in some cases leading to torsades de pointes–type ventricular tachycardia. Drugs in all categories may have other effects that may promote cardiac arrhythmias as an undesired and often unpredicted consequence.

Take, for example, the term *antiarrhythmic drug*. This term is ubiquitous and is the heading used for relevant chapters in virtually all standard textbooks of medicine and pharmacology. The heading encompasses drugs used to treat cardiac electrical instability, primarily tachycardias. The most widely used classification schema (the Vaughan Williams system) for these cardiac drugs is given in Table 9.1, with some specific examples.

The problem with the word *antiarrhythmic* is that it creates an expectation that such drugs will actually have the effect of treating an arrhythmia, resulting in a therapeutic outcome. However, a major finding over the past few decades is that these drugs may be completely ineffective in treating a given arrhythmia. More concerning is that in a small but clinically very important subset of patients, use of these drugs may actually create or induce a *new* arrhythmia, which may prove life-threatening or worsen the very arrhythmia that one is attempting to treat. These paradoxically negative effects are referred

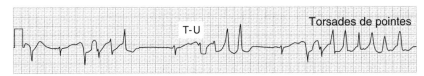

FIGURE 9.1   Proarrhythmic effects of a Class IC "antiarrhythmic" drug.

to as *proarrhythmia* (Figure 9.1). Sometimes they result in iatrogenic sudden cardiac death.

For example, consider the use of oral drugs used to either convert atrial fibrillation or atrial flutter to sinus rhythm, or to maintain sinus rhythm following electrical or pharmacological cardioversion. Drugs used for this purpose fall into several categories based on selected aspects of their mechanisms of activity: class IA (e.g., quinidine, procainamide, disopyramide), class IC (e.g., flecainide, propafenone), and class 3 (e.g., sotalol, amiodarone/dronedarone, dofetilide). However, each agent carries a small but important risk of proarrhythmic toxicities in certain populations and may only be effective in a small set of carefully selected patients.

Most dramatically, drugs in the class IA and IC categories may promote prolongation of repolarization, inducing an acquired type of long QT pattern (see also Chapter 1). In some subjects, when this effect is pronounced, the associated inhomogeneities and instabilities of repolarization may result in the initiation of torsades de pointes, a type of polymorphic ventricular tachycardia (Figure 9.1). In other patients, the drugs (e.g., flecainide) may transform nonsustained ventricular tachycardia into a sustained and potentially lethal version.

Yet use of the term *antiarrhythmic drug* is a historical one and creates the expectation of a consistent pharmacological effect; it would certainly tend to bias clinicians and investigators against the possibility that such drugs might be harmful. A more neutral term would have been *cardiac electrophysiologically active agents*, which indicates that these drugs may alter certain properties of heart tissue via direct and indirect effects but does not create a potentially misleading impression of therapeutic efficacy.

SEMANTIC BIAS AND TARGETED THERAPIES

A second example of semantic bias is the ubiquitous use of the word *target*. The molecular era in medicine has given rise to many exciting approaches to understanding disease pathophysiology (via genes, micro RNAs, and proteins, to name a few) and the expectation that altering these discrete molecular components may have reliable therapeutic effects. This approach to pharmacology is generally referred to as *targeted medicine*, a type of military or sports analogy suggesting that if you hit a target by blocking it or enhancing its function, depending on the circumstance, you will positively affect disease progression and improve outcomes.

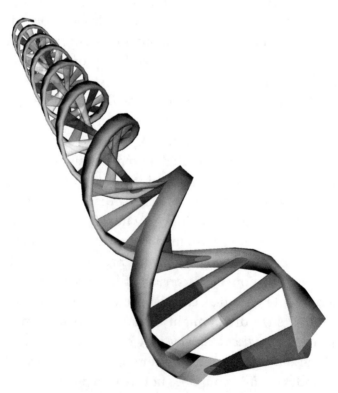

Spirals of life: Where else is bio-information encoded?

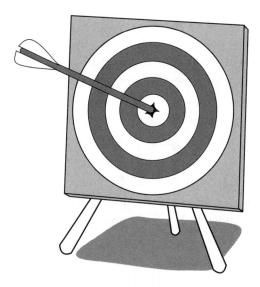

What is the target in a nonlinear system?

Indeed, virtually all of contemporary drug discovery connects with the notion of targeted therapy. The likelihood that you will sit through a grand rounds or seminar presentation in a field of medicine related to drug development and not hear the word *target* is close to zero. What, then, is the problem with the notion of a target? The term is a contemporary version of the classic idea of a *magic bullet* that informed the historically rewarding search for antimicrobial therapy in previous generations. The first use of the term in this context is credited to the great German scientist Paul Ehrlich (1854–1915), cowinner of the 1908 Nobel Prize in Physiology or Medicine:

> If we picture an organism as infected by a certain species of bacterium, it will . . . be easy to effect a cure if substances have been discovered which have a specific affinity for these bacteria and act . . . on these alone . . . while they possess no affinity for the normal constituents of the body . . . such substances would then be . . . magic bullets.

However, even in the therapy of bacterial infections, the notion of a magic bullet sometimes backfires, since such agents give rise to drug-resistant organisms that can be the source of extraordinary harm. In microbiology, the bacteria "learn" to dodge the magic bullets by evolutionary inventiveness. A single staphylococcal organism may not be very adaptive against methicillin. But colonies of bacteria that can reproduce every 20 minutes are brilliantly creative, and multi-drug resistance is a marker of their "genomo-societal" plasticity and reorganizational skills. As a consequence, when an initial bacteriological exam from a patient hospitalized in the United States today demonstrates evidence of gram-positive cocci in clusters, suspicion of methicillin-resistant *Staphylococcus aureus* (MRSA) is so high that it leads to empirical treatment with IV vancomycin (or other agents, such as linezolid), unless subsequent antibiotic sensitivity testing indicates susceptibility to beta-lactam antibiotics.

What are the factors that have thwarted the search for targets in the current molecular era where human cells are the focus? Several basic but sometimes overlooked aspects of biology can be implicated:

- Biological systems are networks, which by definition have interconnected components.
- The crosstalk between these components incorporates both negative (inhibitory) and positive (excitatory) feedback.
- The stimulus–response profiles of these biological components are typically not proportional (i.e., they are not linear).
- Networks, like trees, function over multiple scales of space and time. Local effects may percolate across scales, creating far-field effects. These "off-camera" effects will not be apparent in typical experiments that focus on a very limited view of the system.

Complex Systems and New Mechanisms

These principles, deriving from the contemporary theory of complex systems, underlie the *law of unintended consequences*. Basically, this principle means that in a complex system unexpected things happen and that causality often appears to break down, at least linear causality (domino effects, where $A \rightarrow B \rightarrow C$). Instead of a predictable cascade of events, various types of nonlinear causality occur, so that small changes, sometimes at the amplitude of molecular "noise," can have disproportionate (positive or negative) effects. Micro- or macroscopic changes can alter the entire appearance of a system (qualitative effects emerging from quantitative changes).

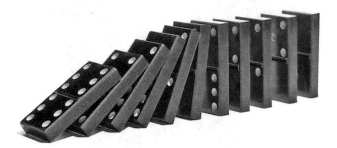

Linear causality and serial collapse of dominos.

Emergent, nonlinear effects are far more common in medicine than one might imagine. For example, a small effective change in drug dose (e.g., of bupropion for depression) might cause a seizure—a dramatic type of abrupt, nonlinear change. Or a premature infant might develop a prolonged pause in breathing (apnea) for no identifiable reason. Changes of this type are reminiscent of *phase changes* in the physical world, where a minuscule fraction of a degree shift can change liquid water to ice, and vice versa. Although we readily accept the scientific basis of such phase changes in our physical environment, doctors and physiologists rarely list them in mechanistic discussions of biological causation.

Is the world of biomedicine linear (such as the domino effect mentioned above) or nonlinear? In a linear world, simple rules → simple behaviors. Things add up and the principle of superposition reigns. There is proportionality of input/output. There is high predictability and no surprises if you have the blueprint. In a nonlinear world, simple rules can lead to complex behaviors, small change may induce huge effects, low predictability and anomalies abound; the whole is qualitatively different from the sum of its parts (Figure 9.2).

Although the concept of nonlinearity may appear esoteric and largely irrelevant in the practical "bottom line" world of the wards, it is actually much closer to our daily lives than you might think. The

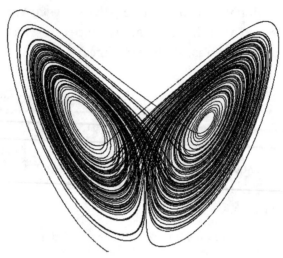

FIGURE 9.2   Lorenz attractor (butterfly effect). Small changes in the initial conditions can have major effects on the long-term trajectories of certain nonlinear systems.

notion of nonlinearity is, in fact, contained in figures of speech that we hear and use almost every day. These include "the straw that broke the camel's back"; "the law of unintended consequences," cited above; "the whole is greater than the sum of the parts"; and "life is a game of inches" (or perhaps angstroms).

As an example of the perils of assuming linear causation in a nonlinear world (or a system governed by nonlinear mechanisms) consider Figure 9.3, a graphical summary of the fluctuations in some variable, such as relative changes in blood pressure over time. The graph shows a complex pattern of variations, punctuated with a bizarre sequence of periodic oscillations and abrupt changes. What would be your hypothesis about the mechanism of these changes in dynamics? You would probably suppose that they represent some process that is being perturbed by stimuli of different types or magnitudes.

What may surprise you is that this output actually arises from a system in which none of the control mechanisms is changing. The *intermittency* or *volatility* that can arise out of the intrinsic dynamics without any change in the control parameters is one of the most

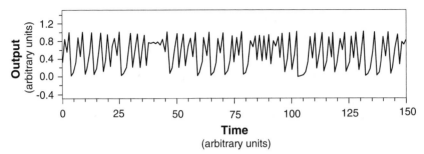

FIGURE 9.3 Example of complex fluctuations in the output behavior of a model system that is governed by nonlinear equations. What makes this example remarkable is the fact that the system is "free-running" and none of the control parameters have been changed. The word *nonlinear* rarely if ever appears in the indexes of physiology or clinical texts, although all biological systems are nonlinear. Our clinical instinct, seeing these kinds of variations, is to impute changes in one or more of the control parameters. However, the scientific experiment (a model simulation here) pulls the rug out from under our "linear" intuitions and traditional notions of causality.

surprising properties of nonlinear systems. The fact that a system that is nonlinear can exhibit changes of this type runs counter to some of our major assumptions of causality. Indeed, it wreaks havoc with them. When we observe qualitative and quantitative changes in the output of any system, we are taught to infer perturbations. But this is not necessarily the case. The extent to which such intermittency occurs in biological systems, which are inherently nonlinear, is unknown. The fact that such behaviors are built into the equations that govern complex systems makes this "strangeness" more likely than not.

What we do know is that current mechanistic models for explaining how drugs affect real-world systems are woefully inadequate. The "evidence" is the number of completely unexpected, usually negative (off-target) effects that are not anticipated in the pharmacological design phase and not detected by conventional drug safety assays.

OFF-TARGET EFFECTS

The term *off-target effects* describes the fact that pharmacological agents frequently have actions that are not predicted by simple cause-and-effect diagrams and mechanisms. Thus, a drug might "hit its target" but have other negative effects that seem to overwhelm the positive effects. For example, some drugs have been withdrawn from the market because of risks to patients, often prompted by unexpected adverse effects that were not detected during phase III clinical trials and were only apparent from postmarketing surveillance data from the wider patient community.

Meridia (sibutramine): Market Withdrawal Due to Risk of Serious Cardiovascular Events

[Posted 10/08/2010]

AUDIENCE: Primary Care, Consumers

ISSUE: Abbott Laboratories and FDA notified healthcare professionals and patients about the voluntary withdrawal of Meridia (sibutramine), an obesity drug, from the U.S. market because of clinical trial data indicating an increased risk of heart attack and stroke.

BACKGROUND: Meridia was approved November 1997 for weight loss and maintenance of weight loss in obese people, as well as in certain overweight people with other risks for heart disease. The approval was based on clinical data showing that more people receiving sibutramine lost at least 5 percent of their body weight than people on placebo who relied on diet and exercise alone. FDA has now requested market withdrawal after reviewing data from the Sibutramine Cardiovascular Outcomes Trial (SCOUT). SCOUT is part of a postmarket requirement to look at cardiovascular safety of sibutramine after the European approval of the drug. The trial demonstrated a 16 percent increase in the risk of serious heart events, including non-fatal heart attack, non-fatal stroke, the need to be resuscitated once the heart stopped, and death, in a group of patients given sibutramine compared with another given placebo. There was a small difference in weight loss between the placebo group and the group that received sibutramine.

RECOMMENDATION: Physicians are advised to stop prescribing Meridia to their patients, and patients should stop taking this medication. Patients should talk to their health care provider about alternative weight loss and weight loss maintenance programs.

Source: U.S Food and Drug Administration (http://www.fda.gov/safety/ medwatch/safetyinformation/safetyalertsforhumanmedicalproducts/ ucm228830.htm)

A tenet of cardiovascular-targeted pharmacology has been that agents that could elevate high-density lipoprotein (HDL, dubbed "good cholesterol" in the popular press) should be beneficial. A promising target should be inhibition of the enzyme cholesteryl ester transfer protein, which normally conveys cholesterol from the high-density lipoprotein (HDL) molecules to very low-density lipoprotein molecules (VLDL or LDL, the latter dubbed "bad cholesterol"). In early preclinical and clinical studies, inhibition of this process with the agent *torcetrapib* resulted in both augmented HDL levels and decreased LDL levels, a "two-fer" combination that should have been powerfully beneficial according to the underlying mechanistic models of atherosclerosis. However, in what is widely acknowledged as a catastrophic failure of the pharmaceutical industry, a large phase III double-blind randomized control trial of the drug was abruptly halted in December 2006. At the advice of the Data Safety Monitoring Board, this study, involving about 15,000 subjects, was halted due to higher all-cases mortality and major adverse cardiovascular events in the torcetrapib arm. What caused the off-target effects that, most important, were clinically harmful and also scuttled a multibillion-dollar investment, and years of well-intentioned work remain incompletely understood.

More recently (May 2011), another large multicenter study designed to test the hypothesis that raising HDL cholesterol in high-risk subjects would lower major cardiovascular events was terminated prematurely. This clinical trial, conducted under the auspices of the National Heart Lung and Blood Institute of the NIH, was ambitiously called AIM-HIGH (Atherothrombosis Intervention in Metabolic Syndrome with Low HDL/High Triglyceride and Impact on Global Health Outcomes). Study participants were administered standard lipid-lowering therapy with simvastatin 40 mg/day, and then randomly assigned to receive either extended-release niacin 1500 to 2000 mg/day or placebo. In the first year of the trial, the simvastatin dose could be adjusted, or a second LDL cholesterol–lowering drug, ezetimibe 10 mg, which decreases intestinal cholesterol absorption, could be added, to achieve the *target* LDL cholesterol goal of 40 to 80 mg/dL. The AIM-HIGH trial was stopped 18 months early due to the lack of added benefit on cardiovascular risk reduction in the extended-release niacin plus simvastatin treatment group over simvastatin alone.

Of note, this failure to improve outcomes occurred despite the finding that participants who took high-dose extended-release niacin and statin treatment had increased HDL cholesterol and lowered triglyceride levels compared to participants who took a statin alone (i.e., the targeted biochemical changes were achieved but the clinical outcomes were not). In addition, a small unexplained increase in the rate of ischemic stroke was noted in the simvastatin plus extended-release niacin group compared to the simvastatin-alone group.

The recurrent findings of studies in which producing a desired biochemical effect do not necessarily reduce the risk of a given disease and may even be associated with adverse effects is deconstructing our fundamental notions about targeted drug therapy. Furthermore, these counterintuitive findings support the cautionary clinical principle that identifying a biomarker of health or disease risk (e.g., high or low HDL) does not necessarily mean that drugs which move that biomarker in a desired direction will, themselves, be associated with positive outcomes.

Off-target effects raise deep questions about our understanding of the molecular pathophysiology of many diseases. These questions are generated by discrepancies between the anticipated vs. actual effects of a growing number of pharmacological agents. For example, bevacizumab, a monoclonal antibody, was developed to treat a number of cancers due to its angiogenesis-blocking effects, mediated by binding to a vascular endothelial growth factor (VEGF-A). However, major side effects have included gastrointestinal viscus perforations, bleeding diatheses, and posterior reversible encephalopathy syndrome. On June 29, 2011, the FDA formally removed bevacizumab (Avastin) for use in metastatic breast cancer, but the drug is still used in selected other malignancies.

Another notable example of off-target effects pertains to the safety of the thiazolindedione, rosiglitazone (Avandia), which has been widely used in the therapy of type II diabetes mellitus. The putative therapeutic effect is related to increasing sensitivity of adipose cells to insulin by binding to one of a class of molecules known as peroxisome proliferator-activated receptors (PPARs). The question that has aroused debate—and in 2010 led to restrictions on its use in the U.S. and its withdrawal in Europe—is whether it has the unexpected effect of causing myocardial infarction and increasing the risk of heart failure. Table 9.2 is a list of initially-approved drugs that were subsequently withdrawn by the FDA between 2000 and 2011.

Students and attendings are encouraged to survey some of the drugs in use and determine to what extent the brand name of the

TABLE 9.2   Notable Drug Withdrawals in the United States 2000–2011

Name	Year	Risk(s)
Troglitazone (Rezulin)	2000	Hepatotoxicity
Alosetron (Lotronex)	2000	Potentially fatal complications of constipation; reintroduced in 2001 on a restricted basis
Cisapride (Propulsid)	2000	Withdrawn in many countries because of the risk of cardiac arrhythmias
Phenylpropanolamine (Propagest, Dexatrim)	2000	Stroke in women under 50 years of age when taken at high doses (75 mg twice daily) for weight loss
Trovafloxacin (Trovan)	2001	Liver failure
Cerivastatin (Baycol, Lipobay)	2001	Rhabdomyolysis
Rapacuronium (Raplon)	2001	Fatal bronchospasm
Rofecoxib (Vioxx)	2004	Myocardial infarction/stroke
Hydromorphone, extended release (Palladone)	2005	Accidental overdose when administered with alcohol
Pemoline (Cylert)	2005	Hepatotoxicity
Ximelagatran (Exanta)	2006	Hepatotoxicity
Rimonabant (Accomplia)	2006	Severe depression and suicide
Pergolide (Permax)	2007	Heart valve damage
Tegaserod (Zelnorm)	2007	Cardiovascular ischemic events, including heart attack and stroke
Aprotinin (Trasylol)	2008	Complications or death
Efalizumab (Raptiva)	2009	Progressive multifocal leukoencephalopathy
Sibutramine (Reductil/ Meridia)	2010	Increased cardiovascular risk and minimal efficacy
Gemtuzumab ozogamicin (Mylotarg)	2010	Fatal toxicity, veno-occlusive disease, and no additional benefit in treating acute myelogenous leukemia
Drotrecogin alfa (Xigris)	2011	No benefit in treatment of sepsis

drug is an attempt to create demand and deemphasize potential side effects. As a hypothetical example: Just because a drug is poetically branded (fictitiously) as "Calmitrol" does not always make it anxiolytic or beneficial in other ways.

SEMANTIC BIOCHEMICAL BIAS

An interesting and more subtle variation on the theme of semantic traps is the way that scientists refer to molecules. Sometimes this everyday naming creates a mechanistic bias that implies one major mode of action, when the effects may be much more diverse. Often, names for physiological signaling mediators are based on the context of their initial discovery. A good example is the hypothalamic peptide arginine vasopressin, which is a hormone with multiple activities and functions. This name implies that it is primarily a vasoconstrictor. Yet it is also the antidiuretic hormone and has a number of important central nervous system actions. Further, it is structurally related to oxytocin.

Another example is the hormone cholecystokinin (CCK), named for its gallbladder-stimulating effects associated with eating, first noted in dogs. However, the effects of this polypeptide, dubbed for its gastrointestinal effects, appear to be manifold. CCK receptors are widespread in the central and peripheral nervous system, and an "anti-opioid" effect has been reported.

Such pleiotropy of effect is not unique to CCK and raises the question of whether the same agonist is interacting with different receptors in different organs, or whether the effects on identical receptors are context dependent and whether the same hormones can function as part of different networks in different organs. More than likely, if CCK had been discovered first in the central nervous system, the hormone would bear a different name. Pleiotropic effects are not unique to endogenous compounds. Several drugs are now being used to treat different, if not altogether unrelated conditions from those they were initially designed to treat (Table 9.3). Indeed, not all side effects may be adverse. A number of these "on (a new) target" side effects are shown in the table.

TABLE 9.3   Changes in Drug Targets

Drug	Initially Prescribed to Treat	Now Used to Treat
Amiodarone	Angina pectoris	Maintenance and restoration of sinus rhythm in atrial fibrillation and atrial flutter
Finasteride	Benign prostatic hyperplasia*	Alopecia in men
Lithium	Gout	Bipolar disorder
Mexiletine	Ventricular arrhythmia (class IB antiarrhythmic)*	Neuropathic pain; weakness in myotonic dystrophy
Sildenafil	High blood pressure	Erectile dysfunction; pulmonary artery hypertension

*Still an approved indication.

HOMEOSTASIS REVISITED

Homeostasis is one of the most widely used terms in biomedicine. A PubMed search of this term at the time of this writing reveals over 160,000 entries. The term has become synonymous with regulation at both the large-scale (physiologic) and small-scale (molecular) levels. *Homeostasis* refers to the notion that healthy systems are self-regulated to maintain a constancy of output, sometimes analogized to an "equilibrium-like" state. The term was coined by a famous Harvard Medical School physiologist, Walter B. Cannon, M.D., and first published in 1929. Dr. Cannon was a remarkable scientist who made numerous seminal contributions to physiology and medicine. He was also a person of extraordinary integrity and generosity.

Two key facets of the contemporary notion of homeostasis are (1) that physiological variables such as heart rate, blood pressure, blood glucose, body temperature, and pH must be maintained within a set range of values (they play "in bounds") and (2) that the underlying control mechanisms act to smooth out variations in these variables so as to maintain a relatively constant state. Thus, physiological control is analogious to the regulation of temperature in the room (or perhaps airplane) in which you are sitting. If the temperature goes above a given set point, cooling occurs to bring it down, and if it goes down below a certain value, warming occurs. In engineering terms, this machine-like type of control is referred to as a "servomechanism." Cannon made numerous contributions to experimental physiology and medicine. His elucidation of the concept of *homeostasis* had its roots in the nineteenth-century theory of the interior milieu of cells proposed by the preeminent French physiologist Claude Bernard (1813–1878). As discussed here, the concept of homeostasis has been taken too literally to mean that healthy physiological systems actually seek constancy. However, medical students are forever in Cannon's debt for a separate reason—he advocated the use of the case method, supplanting the tedious tradition that prevailed well into the twentieth century of teaching medicine via textbooks, not patients.

> **PHYSIOLOGICAL REVIEWS**
> Vol. IX   JULY, 1929
> **ORGANIZATION FOR PHYSIOLOGICAL HOMEOSTASIS**
> **WALTER B. CANNON**

The original description of homeostasis.

IS THE BODY A SERVOMECHANISM TYPE OF MACHINE?

The two basic principles behind the idea of the body as a servomechanism are:

- The importance of autoregulatory mechanisms to keep variables "in bounds" (not controversial)
- The notion of "constant," "single steady-state," or "equilibrium-like" conditions (Figure 9.4)

The notion of servomechanistic control—the body as a "well-tuned" machine—is deeply embedded in our medical culture. From one perspective, the notion of *autoregulation* is clearly intuitive and essential and is validated by careful observation. Physiological systems do contrive to keep variables "in bounds." For example, blood glucose normally does not get too high or too low (even right after a meal or a prolonged overnight fast), and the same goes

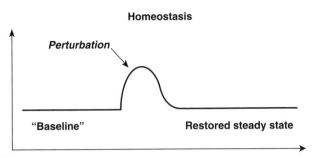

FIGURE 9.4   Homeostasis: Constancy as the "wisdom of the body."

for a myriad of other biochemical measures that have well-defined ranges. The *homeostatic regulation* of serum glucose in response to the stresses of fasting and eating forms the basis of the standard glucose tolerance test.

So, from what perspective does homeostasis need to be reconsidered? The answer comes from recent studies that show that physiological systems, before and after perturbations, do not settle down to a constant state. Indeed, healthy systems under spontaneous free-running conditions normally demonstrate a good deal of "play" in which the variables fluctuate in complex fashion from one instant to the next. Furthermore, these fluctuations, although often subtle, do not simply represent measurement error or random biological "noise."

A good example is the healthy heartbeat. A widely held tenet of physiology is that the normal heartbeat is almost metronomically regular. The idea that you can literally set your watch by the regularity of a resting heartbeat is immortalized by the report of Galileo using his own pulse to time the pendular swinging of the chandelier in the Cathedral of Pisa in 1583. Over 400 years later, this assumption is conveyed in a more mundane way by the ubiquitous clinical designation "RSR," standing for "regular sinus rhythm" to describe the normal ECG. However, consider a lead II rhythm strip (Figure 9.5) from a healthy young woman with an "average" heart rate of 66 bpm. As shown, the heart rate is far from regular, exhibiting changes in rate, due to the changes in vagal tone associated with respiratory phase shifts between inspiration and expiration.

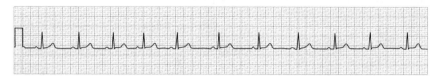

FIGURE 9.5 Rhythm strip (lead II) from the ECG of a healthy, 27-year-old female. Ten seconds of data are shown. Note the prominent variability in the instantaneous rate, ranging from about 60 to 80/min when measured on a beat-to-beat basis. This variability is due to physiological respiratory sinus arrhythmia, which in turn is associated with changes in vagal tone modulation of the sinus node that occur during inspiration (increasing heart rate) and expiration (decreasing heart rate). In addition to these respiratory-related changes, the healthy heartbeat, even at rest, shows highly complex fluctuations. Courtesy of the ECG Wave-Maven site (http://ecg.bidmc.harvard.edu).

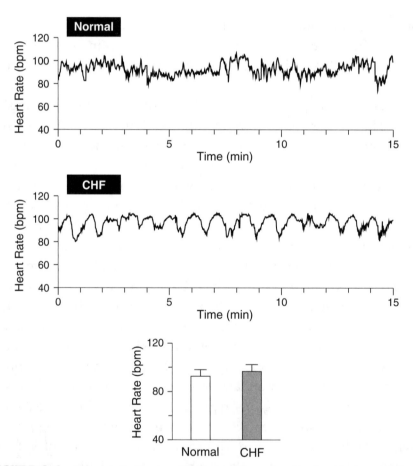

FIGURE 9.6 Heart rate time series in health and with chronic heart failure. The two signals have similar means and variances but very different dynamics. Which is more complex?

Similarly, Figure 9.6 represents the beat-to-beat variability in two subjects, one with a healthy heart and one with heart failure. What is different between the two? As you will see, although their rates are nearly identical, the interbeat variation in the normal heart is much more pronounced than that in the failing heart. Indeed, this plasticity in variation is—you may be surprised to learn—a marker of health.

MINI-SUMMARY

- Students and seasoned clinicians alike need to be aware of a subtle type of semantic bias that has largely escaped notice due to an overly linear view of causality, privileging the notion of isolated "targets."
- Medical terms create expectational biases. For example, just because a drug is called an antiarrhythmic agent doesn't mean that it makes cardiac rhythm disturbances better. It may have no effect or may even cause sudden cardiac arrest and death (proarrhythmia).
- Modern medicine is geared toward curing disease by affecting molecular targets. But keep in mind that medical systems are nonlinear and that targeted interventions may backfire or misfire. Off-target effects are more the rule than the exception. The classic notion of homeostasis (constancy is the wisdom of the body) may need to be revised.
- In all likelihood, a drug that your patient is taking will be discovered to have a previously unknown adverse effect. Some drugs will be taken off the market as a result—be on the lookout for such unreported or underreported toxicities. Yours may be the first (index) report.

CHAPTER 10

SOME SECOND OPINIONS: OUTLIERS, HOOFBEATS, AND SUTTON'S (FLAWED) LAW

Simplicity is the highest goal, achievable when you have overcome all difficulties. After one has played a vast quantity of notes and more notes, it is simplicity that emerges as the crowning reward of art.

—FRÉDÉRIC CHOPIN (1810–1849)

My music aspires to be complex, never complicated.

—MAURICE RAVEL (1875–1937)

Everything should be made as simple as possible, but not simpler.

—ALBERT EINSTEIN (1879–1955)

The purpose of this chapter is to convey some additional considerations that inform and misinform aspects of the way in which even experienced clinicians think about data. Students and their attendings need to be aware of these. A unifying theme is "the observed vs. the (un)expected."

Becoming a Consummate Clinician: What Every Student, House Officer, and Hospital Practitioner Needs to Know, First Edition.
Ary L. Goldberger and Zachary D. Goldberger.
© 2012 Wiley-Blackwell. Published 2012 by John Wiley & Sons, Inc.

OUTLIERS: CLUES OR RUSE?

Not uncommonly when reviewing clinical data, you will note that a given laboratory value (e.g., low serum sodium) or finding from the clinical examination ("loud S3" gallop in a healthy middle-aged man) does not make sense. For example, the diagnoses under consideration do not account for hyponatremia, or the patient does not have heart failure and thus should not have this type of mid-diastolic filling sound. These are examples of findings that appear to be misfits.

Findings that lie outside the expected range for a given context are sometimes labeled *outliers*. They are *symmetry breakers* or pieces of puzzles that have no apparent place. Outliers make clinical diagnoses even trickier and more difficult than they are inherently. Outliers may be time- and cost-consuming distractions that create unnecessary anxiety, yet they may also be real clues to a deeper puzzle than the one being considered.

At least three classes of clinical outliers can be identified:

1. Specimen acquisition, processing, or laboratory errors: machine failure, collection or processing artifacts, (e.g., hemolysis leading to "hyperkalemia"), machine error, and transcribing error, among others.
2. Real values or findings that sometimes give an important clue to a missed diagnosis or help in reconsidering the "conventional wisdom" for a patient.
3. Unexplained findings that should be flagged for follow-up.

An important role for students lies in the systematic review of their patients' charts and the identification of apparent outliers. In the first example cited above, it might turn out that the serum sodium or potassium is erroneous. The error could arise for a number of reasons:

- *Statistical*: the more tests ordered, the higher the likelihood that one is in an abnormal range
- *Mix-up in reporting*: right value but wrong patient
- *Lab error*: wrong value but right patient

- *Processing error*: spuriously high potassium due to hemolysis of red cells (labs usually report evidence of this)

In the second example, perhaps the "S3 gallop" was actually a misinterpreted extra-cardiac sound due to rubbing skin or clothes against a stethoscope. What appeared to be an S3 gallop may actually have been a widely and fixed split S2 due to an atrial septal defect, an opening snap due to mitral stenosis, or a pericardial friction rub sequence simulating an S3.

On the other hand, the finding of apparently profound hyponatremia might be entirely correct—that is, not a lab error, a clinical mix-up, or a spurious value—but is due to a major condition that had not been noted or considered. For example, the patient might have the syndrome of inappropriate diuretic hormone secretion (SIADH) due to a tumor or might have adrenal insufficiency (Addison's disease). Alternatively, the finding (e.g., a sodium of 132 mEq/L) could just be a puzzle—not an apparent error but at the same time not a finding that presents a directional clue. Or the finding could be an "artifact" due to another important abnormality such as hyperlipidemia, which might affect the automated measurement of sodium concentration. Repeating outlier tests is advised.

In the second example, perhaps the so-called "S3 gallop" was actually a misinterpreted extra-cardiac sound due to the rubbing of skin or clothes against your stethoscope. Another possibility is that the S3 gallop might be a real and important pathologic finding due to the unsuspected presence of a dilated, restrictive or hypertrophic cardiomyopathy that is first detected by your keen ear and overlooked by previous physicians, including the current attending. (In a young athletic person, an S3 gallop may be a physiologic finding.)

Or what appeared to be an S3 gallop may have actually been a real auscultatory finding, timed to simulate a mid-diastolic filling sound. The differential diagnosis includes an S2 with wide, fixed splitting due to an atrial septal defect, a widely but physiologically split S2 due to right bundle branch block, an opening snap due to mitral stenosis, a "tumor plop" due to a left atrial myxoma, or part of a three-component pericardial friction rub sequence. Maybe another auscultator was hearing an S1-mitral prolapse click-S2 sequence and misinterpreting it as an S1-S2-S3. How could you help distinguish these possibilities at the bedside (before ordering an echocardiogram)?

As emphasized in Chapter 3, you can lower the probability of laboratory outliers that may create needless distractions with costly consequences by only ordering tests that will affect patient care, are germane to differential diagnoses, and are related to some clinical hypothesis that you are testing.

EQUINE HOOFERS AND BANK LARCENY: TIME TO RETIRE TWO OUTMODED CLINICAL "PEARLS"?

Here's a test: See how long you can go during attending rounds and related medical conferences without hearing reference to one of these two aphorisms:

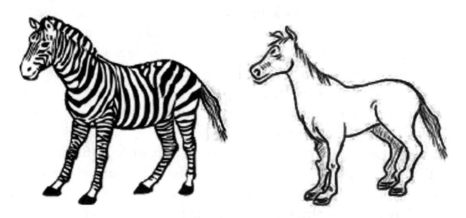

Those hoofbeats: Zebra or horse?

- "When you hear hoofbeats, think of horses, not of zebras."
- "Go where the money is" (referred to as *Sutton's law*).

The prediction here is that within a month you will hear one or both of these statements made by attendings or house staff. In our opinion, they (the sayings, not the attendings) have become dusty, losing their novelty and humorous impact. In short, they are in need of retirement.

ETIOLOGIES AND APPLICATIONS

How to Use Clues

The first (equine) aphorism is used to encourage and sometimes admonish medical students and house staff to think of "common things commonly" and not to run off in search of the obscure and the unlikely—which is wise advice. The saying (which has nothing to do with gallop rhythms) has been attributed to an illustrious scientist, Dr. Theodore E. Woodward, a twentieth-century medical researcher who played a major role in finding cures for typhoid and typhus fever.

So what is wrong with this quote? The answer is that contemporary clinicians are generally pragmatic and cost-conscious. When they see a middle-aged hypertensive patient with bilateral systemic radial artery blood pressures of 170/100 mmHg on repeated recordings, they think of primary (essential hypertension) ahead of secondary hypertension. And in the latter group they think of more common (e.g., renal-based) causes ahead of pheochromocytoma (a "zebra").

However, less common (and especially treatable, reversible, or heritable) causes of disease processes are very impactful. Some of these are relatively rare and others are extremely rare but still of great importance both clinically and in terms of basic disease mechanisms. The National Institutes of Health has a useful website devoted to rare diseases (essentially zebras) at http://rarediseases.info.nih.gov/, as does the National Organization of Rare Diseases (www.rarediseases.org). For U.S. public health classification purposes, a disease is currently considered "rare" if fewer than 200,000 people in the United States have it. There are an estimated 7000 or so such rare diseases, and about 25 million people in the United States have one. So, rare diseases, taken as a group, are not that rare. In the aggregate, they affect up to 8% of the U.S. population.

Hearing hoofbeats usually does mean horses are around the corner, but sometimes they are the sounds of zebras. At other times, what you initially hear as hoofbeats turn out to be sounds of a different nature entirely. Perhaps you will experience the joy of unexpectedly discovering the equivalent of seahorses.

Sutton's (Flawed) Law Revisited

The second aphorism is perhaps the most overcited in medicine and is likely to be misattributed, to boot. The quote is credited to convicted armed bank robber William (Willie) Sutton (1901–1980). Mr. Sutton was also reportedly known by the nicknames "Willie the Actor" and "Slick Willie." Legend has it that he once answered a reporter's question about why he always robbed banks with the response, "Because that's where the money is," thereby immortalizing his name, not so much in the annals of crime but in those of medical diagnostics (see Chapter 6).

Actual credit for incorporating Sutton's "law" into medicine is given to a renowned cardiologist, Dr. William Dock. As described in his *New York Times* obituary at the time of his death at age 91:

"Dr. Dock recalled the reply when, as a professor of medicine at what is now Downstate, he was visiting the Yale Medical School in New Haven and found doctors there puzzled by a mysterious liver ailment in a young girl from Puerto Rico.

Taking note of where she had lived, Dr. Dock suspected that she was afflicted with schistosomiasis, a parasitic disease common in Puerto Rico. Instead of the usual diagnostic routine of expensive blood tests and special x-rays that might have pointed to bad liver function in the patient but still not have pinpointed the cause, he recommended that a small sample of liver tissue be taken for examination.

The biopsy disclosed no abnormalities in the liver, but a medical student who examined the tissue detected the tiny eggs of a schistosome parasite, confirming Dr. Dock's diagnosis. Thus was written Sutton's Law, which tells diagnosticians to use the single test most likely to bear fruit before undertaking a series of routine examinations that may do little more than produce red herrings."

In a double irony, Sutton himself later "confessed" that he was not the source of the quote. He claimed that it was the reporter's wording in the 1976 book he coauthored, *Where the Money Was: The Memoirs of a Bank Robber*. Perhaps, as a topping to a career built on unlawful enterprises, he was only having us on by falsely confessing to not authoring what later became known as Sutton's law. The first and last laughs may have been his. No matter. Sutton's so-called "law" is now fully embedded in the parlance of the wards. The basic idea is that doctors should look in the most obvious place with the most straightforward test to make a diagnosis. In other words, don't waste time and effort. Do the single most direct test first.

Putting aside any ethical awkwardness related to canonizing a serial larcenist's motivation as medical maxim, the "law" itself has limited use. First, it is, of course, not a law at all, but a witticism turned aphorism. Second, and most important, what constitutes the most direct approach to diagnosis may be far from straightforward. Dr. Davies and Dr. Finch in Nottingham, UK, have noted that in fever of unknown origin (FUO), "Sutton's apocryphal law, to 'go where the money is,' is not generally helpful when the potential site of the fever remains inapparent and can lead to unnecessary non-invasive or even invasive investigations" (e.g., lymph node or other tissue biopsies).

To be judiciously fair and balanced, we note that some of our colleagues do vouch for the utility of Sutton's "principle." Students and house officers (with appropriate human subject committee approval) can readily go where the money is, metaphorically, and actually test Sutton's law. The gist of a prospective study would be to design a rigorous assessment of what would be a diagnostic test of choice for medical team members involved in the care of patients whose initial diagnosis is not obvious. How much observer variability is there in applying Sutton's law in ordering a definitive test? Alternatively, the study could be done retrospectively using a CPC-type format. Present written case write-ups giving details of patients' initial presentations that were puzzling and then pose a choice of "go-for-the-money" options (including "other").

The connection between Willie Sutton and any law is ironic at best. Mr. Sutton, former denizen of Sing-Sing prison in Ossining,

New York, did, however, say something universally relevant to what you are doing in the medical profession. When asked why he went into his line of "work" despite the fact that it led to long jail sentences and frequently nonremunerative stints, he said it was because he actually loved the job.

MINI-SUMMARY

- Outlier findings make clinical diagnoses even trickier and more difficult than they are inherently because they may be time- and cost-consuming distractions, but may also be real clues to a deeper puzzle than the one being considered.
- Some diseases and syndromes are relatively rare and others are extremely rare ("zebras") but still of great importance both clinically and in terms of disease mechanisms.

CHAPTER 11

A SIXFOLD PATH: FROM DATA TO KNOWLEDGE TO UNDERSTANDING

The teacher is the one who gets the most out of the lessons, and the true teacher is the learner.
—ELBERT HUBBARD (1856–1915), American editor, author, and publisher

If you haven't found something strange during the day, it hasn't been much of a day.
—JOHN ARCHIBALD WHEELER (1911–2008), colleague of Albert Einstein and eminent American physicist who coined the term *black hole*.

In the preceding chapters we have focused on how doctors process and present information and something of how they think about clinical problems. This brief chapter is about specific strategies for learning en route to becoming a medical maestro, a master of multiple knowledge domains, in the postmodern age of data/(mis)information overload (see Introduction).

> *Key Question*: Since meticulously edited, scholarly textbooks are often outdated before they are printed, and online resources are incomplete and often "unvetted," what strategies can you use to enhance your critical learning and get the best of all worlds: print, electronic, and others yet to be invented?

Becoming a Consummate Clinician: What Every Student, House Officer, and Hospital Practitioner Needs to Know, First Edition.
Ary L. Goldberger and Zachary D. Goldberger.
© 2012 Wiley-Blackwell. Published 2012 by John Wiley & Sons, Inc.

We learn in a variety of ways. There is a rich literature on different learning styles. Each of us is thought to have a favored approach: visual, auditory, kinesthetic, and so on. However, notions of different learning styles and the related topic of multiple types of intelligences are not without their controversies. What we would like to emphasize is that clinical medicine is unique in that it requires a bit of each of these styles and probably favors "disciplined eclectics." As you have undoubtedly noticed, instructors tend to be far more limited in their repertory of didactic tools than students are in their stylistic preferences. Regardless of your preference for learning, medicine still requires a rigorous and rapidly expanding curricular foundation, albeit one that is dynamic and self-revising.

How, then, can you cope with the competing demands of knowing the "trees" and also seeing the "forest"? Obviously, no single best answer is reasonable. Those who have gone through medical training are among the savviest at developing well-honed and even physiologically "hypertrophied" learning skills, analogous to athletes.

The following six general strategies may be helpful to you or your medical students regardless of learning style.

THE NAUTILUS AND THE SPIRAL CURVE OF LEARNING

The nautilus shell is a familiar and beautiful spiral object. It is also a useful metaphor for a concept of tiered or layered learning. For most mortals, reading about any topic the first or fifth time is not sufficient

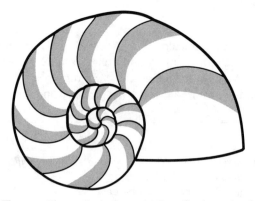

The nautilus spiral: A metaphor for learning?

for mastery. And even if it were, new information will come along to make incomplete or even obsolete what you have just apparently mastered.

A natural impulse is to try to engulf or phagocytose new material in one bite. This approach is usually frustrating and overwhelming. Distention replaces attention. An alternative approach is to encircle, or more figuratively en-spiral, the material you wish to master in wider and wider arcs, like those of the nautilus shell. With each successive spiral you can add and refine information. So the first time you learn about helminthic infections you might get the gist of the major disorders, followed by a wider arc that includes more information (general and specific), and then another arc that subtends the initial ones, leading to a progressively richer knowledge space.

"PATHO-PHYS," NOT "PATHO-LISTS"

Medicine requires the ability to organize and access vast amounts of data in different categories. Little wonder that students and more experienced clinicians are on the lookout for convenient mnemonic devices or other ways of remembering lists. A simple Internet search under this topic will turn up many sites with medical memory aids ("patho-lists"). There is nothing inherently wrong with using such devices. Indeed, we all use mnemonic methods in our daily lives. But in medicine, living by lists has four major limitations:

1. It's usually far easier to remember the acronymic title of the lists (e.g., DEMENTIA for eight common causes of dementia, or PIRATES for seven clinical settings predisposing to atrial fibrillation) than to remember the actual items.

2. The lists are usually incomplete, exceptions being those used to recall the bones of the hand and comparably limited anatomical sets.

3. The lists provide no basic mechanistic understanding; they may be clever and some are memorably risqué, but they have little or nothing to do with the basis of medical knowledge or practice.

4. The lists also discourage thinking about multicause syndromes (e.g., anemia that is due to a combination of blood loss, chronic disease, and hemolysis).

As a case study, consider the differential diagnosis of *hyperkalemia*, a major and life-threatening clinical syndrome:

Mnemonic approach. A number of mnemonics have been proposed for hyperkalemia: miminalistically is A HI K, in which A = acidosis, H = hypoaldosteronism; I = inaccurate lab or inaccurate reading, and K = kidney disease. More ambitious is ALDOSTERONE—you can try to figure this one out for yourself.

Pathophysiologic approach. From a pathophysiological viewpoint, hyperkalemia is related to one and often some combination of three basic processes: (1) decreased renal K^+ excretion, (2) increased extracellular K^+ shifts, and (3) increased K^+ loading. Further, as described in Chapter 6, the first category in virtually every differential diagnosis is "artifact or spurious causes."

Putting it together, for hyperkalemia a reasonable working differential diagnosis for students and non-nephrologists would include five major categories, shown in Exhibit 11.1. with some examples from each category. Note that this pathophysiologic-based list is not meant to be exhaustive but to give a sense about how such differential diagnostic lists can be developed from fundamental principles rather than rote memorization or mnemonic aids.

Note to Attendings: Pathophysiologic-based differential diagnoses are a higher and essential step in developing a deeper understanding of disease processes. For those who have the background (or wish to engage trainees in this effort), going even further back and more deeply to first principles—in this case the basic principles of the regulation of potassium in human physiology—would be a worthy goal and one that would solidify often missing connections between the preclinical and clinical years (see the Introduction).

EXHIBIT 11.1   Pathophysiology of Hyperkalemia, With Examples[a]

Spurious or artifactual
  Lab error
  Fist-clenching effect during blood draw
  Hemolysis of red cells in vitro (usually noted by lab)
  Pseudo-hyperkalemia due to marked thrombocytosis or leukocytosis (leakage of K^+
    in vitro)
Decreased renal K^+ excretion
  Intrinsic renal disease syndromes
  Decreased effective renal perfusion: hypovolemia or heart failure
Aldosterone insufficiency syndromes
  Primary (e.g., Addison's disease)
  Secondary: hyporeninemic hypoaldosteronism (e.g., in diabetic nephropathy)
  Drugs blocking release and/or effect: angiotensin-converting enzyme inhibitors
    and angiotensin II receptor blockers, nonsteroidal anti-inflammatory drugs,
    cyclosporine, spironolactone, eplerenone, triamterene, amiloride
Increased extracellular K^+ shifts
  Acidemia: metabolic or respiratory
  Tissue damage (e.g., with crush injuries, rhabdomyolysis, tumor lysis, accidental
    hypothermia)
  Severe digitalis overdose
  Beta-2 adrenergic blockade (usually mild effects)
  Hyperkalemic periodic paralysis
Excessive potassium loading
  Oral
  Parenteral (intravenous or intramuscular)

[a]This is only a partial list of specific causes under the major headings; after exclusion of spurious and artifactual, decreased renal excretion is the most important category, and multiple factors may coexist (e.g., muscle and renal damage or heart failure, renal disease, and drugs that block aldosterone release or effects).

SALTATION: LEARNING BY LEAPS AND BOUNDS

The term *saltatory* is one you might recall from preclinical lectures on nerve conduction. It has nothing to do with NaCl. Instead, this process relates to rapid propagation of impulses usually along myelinated nerves, in which the impulse appears to hop or jump (hence saltatory, based on the Latin). In this context, the term is used more metaphorically. An effective strategy for learning is to hop among topics from time to time. For example, when you are reading about one topic and a new one comes up, you can briefly jump and learn about a new connection. The very act of making such connections serves at least two functions: (1) it reinforces the material you are learning, and

(2) it opens up new areas for exploration and discovery. This process is very close to the implementation of hypertexting, but not everything you may want to hop to is going to have a hypertext link. Thus, you need to create your own networks, not just use those grooved by the authors of a given document.

To use the preceding example as the initiating point of a free-wheeling saltatory exploration (destination unknown), you might start with the term *hyperkalemia*, which might lead to Addison's disease, which might lead to autoimmune endocrine disorders, which might lead to thyroiditis, and so on. Or from Addison's disease you might segue to disseminated tuberculosis and then to an entirely different set of saltatory docking stations. Using this approach, one could likely crisscross a path of infinite variety, encompassing a textbook of medicine (or perhaps write your own).

SKETCHING: THE ART OF LEARNING MEDICINE

The term *art of medicine* has been supplanted (some would say evicted) in many quarters by a hard-nosed interpretation of the notion of evidence-based medicine (see Chapter 8). Here we are not referring to the art of medicine per se—nuanced, hard-to-quantify knowledge base developed by years of clinical experience. Rather, we literally refer to art in the sense of sketching. To avoid misconception, please note that we are not suggesting that you take art lessons, although art appreciation courses are becoming more common in medical schools lately. What we are proposing is the following rule: The better you can draw it, the better you know it.

Thus, whether you are learning about metabolic pathways, cytoskeletal architecture, ECG waves and patterns related to cardiac electrical activation or the anatomy of the femoral vein and nearby structures, the ability to sketch things out is very helpful in mastering the material. If you can draw it, you are more likely to have mastery of it.

- Can you sketch the right and left subclavian veins and surrounding structures?
- Can you sketch out the pathogenesis of ketosis and dehydration with diabetic ketoacidosis?

- Can you sketch the basic ECG patterns in leads V1 and V6 under normal activation, then left and right bundle branch block, and explain their mechanisms in terms of vectors (arrows)?

A useful extension of this principle, which you may consider as a separate category, is the use of medical mannequins and simulators to practice procedures such as resuscitation, pelvic exams, and subclavian and arterial lines. Hands-on tools are invaluable teaching aids.

MULTISOURCING

Students often want to know what are the best textbooks or best electronic sources for a given subject. Whatever the topic, bear in mind that it is optimally accessed via multiple sources. This is not multitasking but multisourcing. The process of hearing or seeing material from different venues is very powerful. Importantly, it may uncover discrepancies and errors that get perpetuated from one source to the next. Moreover, you should always question the assumptions, overt and hidden, in whatever you read or hear ("find the soft spots") and then attempt to reconfigure the material in your own terms. Reconfiguring information in your own words (and pictures) is a very useful way of figuring out what the terms actually mean, how they are supposed to fit together, and where the incomplete areas and larger gaps are in your understanding. Always try to find something that does not fit (see Chapter 10 on outliers).

TEACHING: THE ESSENTIAL PATH TO LEARNING AND MASTERY

Perhaps the best way to consolidate information, to make it your own, is to teach it to others. Possible audiences include not only students, house staff, and senior colleagues, but also yourself. That statement sounds paradoxic and even absurd: How can you lecture to yourself without acquiring some unwanted *DSM* (Diagnostic and Statistical Manual) characteriological label? One answer is that you can write up lecture notes and prepare e-handouts on any material or topic you are studying. But the process of presenting the material in an interactive way with audience questions is perhaps the most effective means to mastery.

One last word on giving prepared talks: You will earn your audience's eternal gratitude and outshine most of your attendings if you keep in mind the following six guidelines (which are almost never followed in our experience, leaving audiences at best intrigued and at worst bewildered and even annoyed):

1. Always present an outline.
2. Avoid wordy slides—almost all should have relevant graphics.
3. Put material in your own words—avoid hand-me-down slides that you don't edit and, of course, copy-and-pastes from the Internet. (Not that you would even consider doing that.)
4. Never present a graph without defining the axes and identifying the proper units.
5. Always let your audiences know the answers to three questions: (a) What is the state of the art? (b) What are the key controversies? and (c) What are the key unanswered questions, basic and clinical, which are grist for future studies? In many cases, this information is not readily available from textbooks or online sources; attendings and hospital experts will be most helpful. Acknowledge them gratefully!
6. Follow the "10% rule set." However slowly and carefully you present material, your audience will likely follow or recall at best 10% in the short term; similarly, only 10% of what you read or are told on a given clinical subject today will have longer-term validity. These percentages are guestimates.

MINI-SUMMARY

Six methods that are useful in conjunction with traditional approaches to help master concepts are the *nautilus shell* (spiral approach), *saltation* (jumping through interrelated topics), *multisourcing*, creating *pathophysiological outlines* (in place of the usual mnemonic aids), *sketching*, and *teaching*.

CHAPTER 12

WHAT IS DISEASE? WHAT IS HEALTH?

> Doctors are men who prescribe medicines of which they know little, to cure diseases of which they know less, in human beings of whom they know nothing.
>
> —Voltaire (1694–1778)

> To study the phenomenon of disease without books is to sail an uncharted sea, while to study books without patients is not to go to sea at all.
>
> —Sir William Osler (1849–1919)

If you want to win a friendly wager, turn to a fellow student or house officer (or if you have sufficient courage, to one of your attendings), and bet that they cannot readily answer two basic questions: "What is disease?" and "What is health?" Attendings can pose the same query to their students, residents, fellows (especially those who might be a bit overconfident), or even colleagues.

WHAT IS A DISEASE?

Next, if you want to up the ante, ask your colleague not only to define the term *disease* but to distinguish it from *syndrome*. Are the two terms

Becoming a Consummate Clinician: What Every Student, House Officer, and Hospital Practitioner Needs to Know, First Edition.
Ary L. Goldberger and Zachary D. Goldberger.
© 2012 Wiley-Blackwell. Published 2012 by John Wiley & Sons, Inc.

identical? Or is a syndrome one class of disease processes? Further, in what respect is the syndrome of inappropriate antidiuretic hormone secretion related semantically to the posttraumatic stress disorder syndrome?

Consulting the world's leading textbooks of medicine for help with these definitions is problematic—no definitions are given. Neither the contributors to this book nor any of the colleagues we polled can recall any course in medical school where the definitions of disease or disease syndromes, the very basis of our profession, were discussed explicitly.

- Standard dictionary definitions of *disease* consider *conditions of the living body or of one of its parts that impair normal functioning and are typically manifested by distinguishing signs and symptoms.* Synonyms include *malady*, *disorder*, and *pathology*.
- A *syndrome* is defined as *a group of signs and symptoms that occur together and characterize a particular abnormality or condition.*

One obvious problem with the first of these two definitions is that some diseases do not actually impair functioning until a more advanced stage or some threshold is crossed. For example, coronary artery disease is often completely asymptomatic and may produce no evidence of physiological impairment until the person presents with a heart attack or sudden cardiac arrest, possibly resulting in death. In such cases, a person with a clearly demonstrable disease process (in this case, by autopsy evidence) may not even have time to develop sustained symptoms (i.e., chest pressure, shortness of breath, palpitations, etc.), let alone become a patient.

The usual definition of disease also relies on impairment of what is called "normal functioning," creating an endless-loop circularity in which disease is the absence of health and health the absence of disease. An even more subtle problem with the standard definition is illustrated by the following question: Is localized, low-grade in situ cancer of the prostate detected at postmortem examination in an 80-year-old man who dies of a massive stroke a disease, or is it just an incidental finding (see Chapter 3)?

Dr. Judah Folkman and Dr. Raghu Kalluri of Harvard Medical School, in a 2004 article in *Nature*, reviewed data related to a striking observation:

> Many of us may have tiny tumours without knowing it. In fact, autopsies of individuals who died of trauma often reveal microscopic colonies of cancer cells, also known as in situ tumours. It has been estimated that more than one-third of women aged 40 to 50, who did not have cancer-related disease in their life-time, were found at autopsy with in situ tumours in their breast. But breast cancer is diagnosed in only 1% of women in this age range. Similar observations are also reported for prostate cancer in men. Virtually all autopsied individuals aged 50 to 70 have in situ carcinomas in their thyroid gland, whereas only 0.1% of individuals in this age group are diagnosed with thyroid cancer during this period of their life.

In this context, more questions arise: Do such ubiquitous in situ cancers, discovered as "incidental" findings at autopsy, or in biopsy or imaging studies while we are still alive, qualify as diseases? If so, should they be treated? How much harm is done unintentionally by treating abnormalities, even cancers that will have no prognostic impact? On the other hand, how much harm is done by missing subtle, preclinical conditions that fly under the radar of conventional screening?

AGING AND DISEASE

Along a similar line of inquiry, one might ask: Is "physiological aging" a disease? Getting old is, after all, associated with loss of normal, or at least optimal, functioning of multiple organ systems (creatinine clearance, memory, golf putting ability, etc.) and is the source of innumerable complaints (especially about the latter two deficits).* Yet

---

*A syndrome well known to golfers, especially experienced older ones, is an affliction that has been called the "yips," which is characterized by sudden jerky movements, tremors, or freezing when trying to perform a golf shot, notably putting. Current evidence supports the concept that some cases of the yips represent a focal dystonia, the same family of task-specific cramping pathologies that can occur during writing and musical performance.

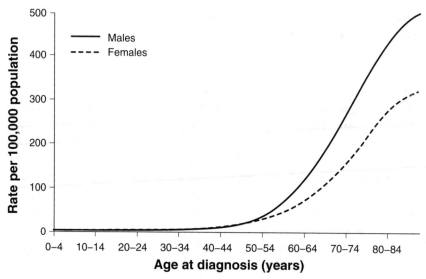

FIGURE 12.1 The rising prevalence of colorectal cancer with advancing age. Adapted from Ballinger AB, Anghiansah C. BMJ. 2007;335:715–718. Reproduced with permission.

physiological (sometimes termed successful or healthy) aging is not considered a disease per se, although many diseases increase markedly in frequency with aging (Figure 12.1). Furthermore, the clinical term *premature aging* implies that aging itself is a pathological or at least a prepathological state.

An emerging area of geriatrics focuses on the *frailty syndrome*, a very common type of pathological aging characterized by a constellation, including weakness, fatigue, weight loss, decreased balance, reduced physical activity, slowed motor processing and performance, social withdrawal, cognitive impairment, and increased vulnerability to stressors. The frailty syndrome (Figure 12.2) is of interest because of its increasing prevalence in the United States and other postindustrial countries, and because it is not a specific disease. Instead, frailty includes markers suggesting a multisystem process that is important because it indicates a statistically significant increase in risk of falls, dementia, heart disease, serious infections, and so on. The approach to the diagnosis and treatment of frailty is challenging contemporary notions of "static biomarkers" (single tests) and also of therapeutic "targets" (magic bullets, discussed in Chapter 10). An important consequence of the concept of frailty as a breakdown of integrative

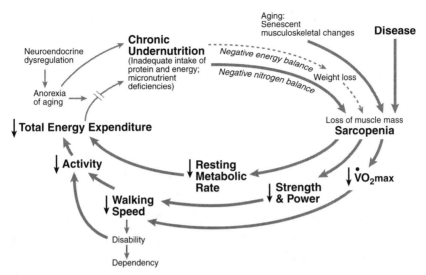

FIGURE 12.2 Frailty is the result of a syndromic set of dynamical processes. From Fried LP et al. J Gerontol A Biol Sci Med Sci. 2001; 56: M146–M156. Reproduced with permission.

function is that its treatment is likely to require multimodal approaches (e.g., exercise, social interactions, osteopenia therapy) rather than a single magic bullet.

PRIMARY DISEASE VS. INADVERTENT INJURY

The dictionary definitions of *disease* and *syndrome* given earlier also fail to distinguish clearly between primary diseases and injuries. A Colles fracture (of the distal radius) impairs functioning and has distinguishing signs and symptoms, but clinicians do not usually consider a bone fracture due to falling off a bicycle or tripping on a niece's rollerblades a disease process. However, if the fracture is associated with some underlying bone impairment, such as osteoporosis, metastatic cancer, multiple myeloma, or osteogenesis imperfecta, the notion of a disease process becomes more relevant and the term *pathologic fracture* is applied. Or, if the precipitating event is a fall due to a syncopal attack from a cardiac arrhythmia or from a seizure, the injury also becomes part of a disease process. Trauma, itself, may also induce a cascade of pathophysiological events involving activation of inflammatory and coagulative systems that may lead to severe sepsis with multiorgan dysfunction syndrome, an all-too-common downward spiral associated with exorbitant mortality in intensive care units.

Additional Questions

- What about the side effects and transient toxicities of drugs that may have therapeutic actions? Are they diseases?
- Is constipation from a calcium-channel blocker, such as vera-pamil, a disease since it impairs intestinal function and produces distinct symptoms?
- Is syncope or even sudden cardiac arrest from the proarrhythmic effects of an antiarrhythmic drug such as quinidine or flecainide a disease?
- Is sickle cell trait a disease, or only if the person becomes symptomatic under unusual stresses related to high-altitude exposure or exhaustive exercise?
- Do other genetic variations, related to DNA or perhaps RNA inhibitors that produce even more subtle structural or metabolic derangements or modifications, constitute diseases?
- What about family and social factors that have a high (statistically significant), but usually nonspecific, correlation with behavioral and physical disorders? Are poverty and homelessness legitimately considered part of disease processes? What about marital divorce? Job stress? War? These terms probably do not appear in the index of the state-of-the-art medical textbook on your desk or e-reader but may well factor into the pathogenesis of your next admission. (They are also rarely, if ever, mentioned in clinical pathological presentations in medical journals or on attending rounds.)

INTERNAL STRESS AND DISEASE: THE CAREGIVER SYNDROME

An important and increasingly recognized link between stress and illness occurs in people, especially family members, who have major responsibility for taking care of others with a chronic illness. The physical and emotional stressors have been associated with major adverse medical consequences, including severe clinical depression, immune dysfunction, premature aging, cardiac disease, and even increased mortality. The term *caregiver syndrome* is used widely now to describe what Dr. Jean Posner, a neuropsychiatrist, has defined as "a debilitating condition brought on by unrelieved, constant caring for a person with a chronic illness or dementia."

The causes of this syndrome challenge conventional notions of mechanisms and are probably multifactorial, including induction or augmentation of neuroautonomic and biochemical alterations that promote a proinflammatory, procoagulative state. The degree to which difficult-to-quantify factors such as physical stress, sleep deprivation, anxiety and guilt, social isolation, and economic hardship play a role is speculative and may vary from one caregiver to another. By its very nature, this syndrome also challenges our target-based, "pharmacocentric" approaches to disease management (Chapter 9). At the very least, clinicians should query patients and their family members about aspects of caregiving roles.

EXTERNAL STRESS AND DISEASE

For a dramatic example of the putative link between stress and pathology, consider this observational case study. A major earthquake struck the Los Angeles Northridge area at 4:31 a.m. on January 17, 1994. This geological event was one of the strongest ever recorded in a major North American metropolis. The earthquake provided a unique opportunity to study the immediate relationship between emotional stress and sudden cardiac death and all-cause mortality. Dr. Jonathan Leor and colleagues at the Good Samaritan Hospital of the University of Southern California reported that the day of the earthquake coincided with a sharp and highly significant (about fivefold) increase in the number of sudden deaths from cardiac causes, spiking from a daily average of 4.6 ± 2.1 in the preceding week to 24 on the day of the earthquake.

Similarly, a significant increase in life-threatening ventricular arrhythmias was reported in patients with implantable cardioverter-defibrillators in the New York City area in the month following the

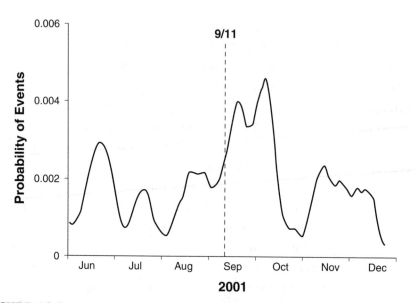

FIGURE 12.3 The day-to-day incidence of ventricular tachyarrhythmia triggering implantable cardioverter-defibrillator (ICD) therapy during an eight-month observation period. Note the substantial spike in event rate in the 30-day period after September 11, 2001. From Steinberg JS, et al. J Am Coll Cardiol. 2004;44:1261–1264. Reproduced with permission.

Al Qaeda terrorist attacks against the United States on September 11, 2001 (see Figure 12.3). What are possible mechanistic connections between stress and sudden death, or stress and the appearance or progression of other disease processes?

The provocative and still controversial *fetal origins of disease hypothesis* stretches our notion of disease still further. The premise is that susceptibility to adulthood cardiovascular disease, insulin resistance, and type 2 diabetes mellitus may be "programmed" in utero in response to fetal undernutrition. This theory is sometimes referred to as the *thrifty phenotype hypothesis.*

DEFINING DISEASE AND HEALTH: ALTERNATIVE APPROACHES

The examples of pathologies noted above, both proven and provocative, uncover limitations in clarifying the definition of disease and suggest the need for other strategies. One reasonable approach to reconsidering what constitutes a disease would be to define it by what it is not: the absence of healthy function in one or more organs or in the system as a whole. However, this strategy also leads to immediate complications. The same textbooks that lack any definition of disease or pathological syndromes also do not offer even a single paragraph, much less a chapter, describing what health is! As stated earlier, one soon becomes knotted in an endless loop in which disease is defined by the absence of health and health by the absence of disease. The standard textbooks do, of course, provide extensive tables with normal limits and ranges for a wide variety of laboratory tests and physiological variables. But tabulated numbers are of very limited value in the overall definition of health.

WHAT IS HEALTH?

Health is one of the most difficult and perhaps most controversial medical concepts to define. To answer this question is not just to engage in a distracting philosophical debate. The entire enterprise of medicine is devoted to curing disease and to restoring and maintaining health. The reflex response that health is simply the absence of disease is neither rigorous nor intuitively satisfying. Defining health by negation, essentially saying that you are "nondiseased," is like calling life the state of being "un-dead." What are the ingredients of health or, even better, of healthy function?

*More than the absence of disease, health is an active dynamical state** *that implies not just physiological functioning of component organs and of the overall organism, but also the integrated ability to cope with a very wide range of often unpredictable intrinsic and extrinsic physical and psychological stresses.* Healthy systems interact both within and without in creative and adaptive ways. In a sense, the healthiest systems are the most supple and resilient. The capacity of a system to cope (its *copability*) is closely related to the reserve of the system (its *capability*).

---

*Dynamical is not a misprint here. Rather it is a term derived from the study of complex systems (Chapter 9) and is different from the term *dynamic*. The latter implies change and variability, but not necessarily a coherent set of mechanisms or a set of governing rules. A dynamical system is one that evolves to some type of rules but may also involve random influences.

IMPLICATIONS: GENERAL AND SPECIFIC

The purpose of this section is not to provide a perfect definition of disease, of disease syndromes, or of health. Consensus on these issues is not likely. The standard dictionary definitions given above, although flawed, are certainly reasonable starting points for discussion, deconstruction, and debate. Most generally, we raise the questions above because they illustrate how ambiguous even the most apparently secure descriptions in medicine are: that is, health vs. disease. As discussed in the Introduction and Chapter 7, ambiguity is a fundamental aspect of medicine and a major motivation for and limitation of *evidence-based medicine*.

Importantly, students of medicine should not grow too reliant on contemporary diagnostic categories, proposed mechanisms of disease, and tests currently available. These key, taken-for-granted elements of the clinical world are all likely to be upgraded, amended, or completely replaced over the years, in some cases beginning tomorrow or even yesterday. More specifically, we do propose two practical suggestions for clinicians.

1. For most conditions, it is more useful and accurate to think about and refer to *disease processes* rather than to diseases. The addition of the word *process* may seem like a small semantic add-on, but it has very important and practical implications. A useful and highly prevalent example is coronary artery disease (CAD) presenting with acute myocardial infarction. This acute coronary syndrome is described more accurately as a disease process that typically has an asymptomatic prodrome, rather than a catastrophic event ("heart attack") appearing suddenly in a person with a perfectly normal cardiovascular system.

In fact, the CAD process usually starts years before an unstable coronary syndrome occurs (acute myocardial infarction, new onset or progressive angina, or even sudden death) and includes a progression of atherogenic stages culminating in a ruptured coronary plaque. The process probably began decades before the presenting problem, in early adolescence or even in childhood in industrialized countries, with the onset of subtle damage (especially due to excess lipids and increased blood pressure) to the coronary artery endothelium. Indeed, Dr. William Aird of Harvard Medical School and his colleagues have proposed that the endothelium itself may constitute a neglected organ system rather than simply comprising a cellular "pavement."

Referring to such pathologies as *disease processes* rather than as *point-like events* also encourages clinicians to include in their pathogenetic discussions important and sometimes modifiable risk factors and contributors that otherwise get marginalized. In the case of CAD, potentially modifiable risk factors include diet, diabetes, hypertension, obesity, dyslipidemias, job stress, and depression.

For community-acquired pneumonia, the risk factors (only some potentially modifiable) include age (the very young or elderly), influenza or other viral syndromes, exposure to infectious agents (e.g., Legionnaire's disease), chronic underlying conditions such as Parkinson's disease or the frailty syndrome, chronic bronchitis, immune dysfunction associated with stress or steroid use, and others.

2. Use the word *syndrome* rather than *disease* to refer to constellations of signs or symptoms that occur together (e.g., posttraumatic stress disorder or heart failure) but do not necessarily share a common cause.

Contrary to common clinical parlance, heart failure is a syndrome and not a disease. Patients typically share common symptoms (fluid retention, dyspnea, fatigue, and exercise limitation) and signs (e.g., resting sinus tachycardia, S3 gallop, basilar lung rales, pedal edema). Their perturbed physiology is marked by a relative decrease in cardiac output, inadequate to meet systemic demands despite normal or increased cardiac filling (diastolic) pressures. However, signing patients in or out of the hospital with just the diagnosis of heart failure is akin to assigning them the diagnosis of "fever."

The obvious follow-up question with the latter diagnosis is, "Fever due to what cause?" If the cause is undetermined and the fever is present for a sufficiently long time, the diagnosis becomes fever of unknown origin (FUO).* Surprisingly, clinicians who would consider a diagnosis of fever to be completely inadequate will use the term *heart failure* without requiring a statement about the likely etiology.

Furthermore, distinct from a specific disease, the heart failure syndrome subtends low output and high output pathophysiologial subvariants, as well as systolic and diastolic subsets, and may itself be the end stage of many specific processes, ranging from CAD, to systemic (essential) hypertension, to cardiomyopathy and valve disease, or often to some combination of these pathologies.

In contrast, application of the term *disease* implies a more consistent set of pathophysiological derangements. For example, hypertensive heart disease is treated as a relatively specific entity that may itself lead to the heart failure syndrome.

SYNDROMES WITHIN SYNDROMES

Even the seemingly "pure" causal example of hypertensive cardiovascular disease leading to heart failure syndrome is not as neat as clinical summaries and some textbooks might suggest. Systemic hypertension is itself a syndrome more than a disease. The most common variant, essential hypertension, is idiopathic and often multifactorial. Renal disease, the other most important cause of systemic hypertension, may be due to renovascular diseases (fibromuscular dysplasia or atherosclerotic disease) or various renal parenchymal diseases.

What about other apparently well-characterized syndromes? Hyponatremia-related syndromes all share one common and obvious feature, a reduction in serum sodium ion concentration. This labora-

*This term actually has objective, albeit somewhat arbitrary and evolving definitions. It was defined initially by Drs. Robert Petersdorf and Paul Beeson at Yale University School of Medicine as the triad of (1) fever higher than 38.3°C (101°F) measured on "several" occasions, (2) persisting without diagnosis for at least 3 weeks, and (3) after at least 1 week of determining an etiology as an inpatient. This is now termed *classic FUO*, due to recent revisions of the definition. Newer criteria call for (1) three outpatient visits or 3 days in the hospital without determining a cause for fever, or (2) 1 week of "intelligent and invasive" ambulatory investigation. What are potential flaws in this newer definition?

tory abnormality (after "correcting" for the degree of hyperglycemia and after excluding spurious causes due to hyperlipidemia, etc.) may in turn be associated with three volemic states: euvolemic, hypervolemic (edematous), and hypovolemic.

However, a major "cause" of the first category of euvolemic hyponatremia is inappropriate ADH secretion, which is a syndrome and not a disease. Furthermore, the different causes of hyponatremia are fundamentally unrelated, such as those associated with heart failure or Addison's disease. Therefore, is hyponatremia really a syndrome or is it a lab abnormality in search of syndromic attachments? Can there be syndromes within syndromes? The closer we get to many syndromes, the less they behave like a *group of concomitant signs or symptoms that characterize a particular abnormality or condition.*

Medical advances also indicate that many conditions that we previously considered to be discrete or monolithic diseases are actually more nonspecific syndromes, with multiple causes and substrates. A good example is atrial fibrillation. Until recently, atrial fibrillation was considered to be a homogeneous entity, at least by ECG criteria. However, rather than a specific cardiac arrhythmia, atrial fibrillation is now being revealed to have a variety of electrophysiological mechanisms (associated with multiple wavelets and/or increased focal atrial automaticity from the pulmonary veins or other areas) and to represent more of a common end-stage dynamic in a variety of settings than a uniquely defined disease. A more refined understanding of this ancient arrhythmia may help develop more appropriate therapies and preventive strategies, ranging from pharmacological to ablational.

A SELF-CHALLENGE

As a useful exercise, readers are encouraged to further examine the dictionary definitions given above and to develop their own conceptual framework for health and disease. Address, for example, the following two questions:

1. Are systemic lupus erythematosus and other idiopathic multisystem immune complex pathologies diseases or syndromes?

2. Is obesity a disease or a syndrome, or neither, unless the patient has some directly related complication, such as a stress fracture, alveolar hypoventilation/sleep apnea, or type 2 diabetes mellitus?

The interwoven processes of constantly rethinking assumptions and researching information are fundamental to practicing medicine successfully, to avoiding potentially lethal errors, and to advancing ways that are both rigorous and compassionate in the inseparable scientifically informed practices of prevention, palliation, and healing.

Clinicians have two major, complementary responsibilities to their patients. We conclude by returning to a central theme of this book, enunciated in the Preface. The successful practice of medicine and the advancement of medical science are rooted in the interwoven processes of constantly rethinking assumptions and researching information. Toward this goal, clinicians have the following two major, complementary responsibilities:

1. To render with compassion and dignity the highest quality, scientifically based care to patients with *diseases* and *traumatic injuries*.
2. To try to preserve and restore *healthy function*.

Yet the definitions of these terms, on which the health care profession is based, remain surprisingly elusive.

MINI-SUMMARY

- Diseases are best conceptualized as processes rather than as discrete events.
- Health is a dynamical state of integrative systems and social functionality, adaptability, and robustness, not simply an aggregate of normal laboratory tests or the absence of disease.
- A key element toward developing medical knowledge and understanding is reworking and reshaping information in your own words, using your own constructs.

BIBLIOGRAPHY AND NOTES

Note 1: The references are intended to be starting points for exploring a vast literature on the different topics covered here. However, we have given preference to those not likely to be in standard medical texts.

Note 2: The University of Massachusetts Medical School in Amherst, Massachusetts, created an innovative "interstitial curriculum" as part of the third-year program that is designed to provide focus on cross-disciplinary topics such interprofessional education, learning communities, and journal club sessions. In contrast, we use the term *interstitial curriculum* in a different context to describe what we consider important aspects of clinical training and practice that are not taught explicitly or do not receive sufficient emphasis in the primary curriculum, potentially leading to an incomplete and frustrating approach to bedside medicine.

Note 3: An intimidating term for "thinking about thinking" is *metacognition*. Since this is meant to be a user-friendly book and since the authors have no philosophical bona fides, we refer interested readers to a growing literature on this subject as applied to philosophy education.

Introduction   Surviving and Thriving in Ward World

Doufas AG, Saidman LJ. The Hippocratic paradigm in medicine: origins of the clinical encounter. Anesth Analg. 2010;110:4–6.

Gleick J. The Information: A History, A Theory, A Flood. New York: Random House, 2011.

Hafferty FW. Beyond curriculum reform: confronting medicine's hidden curriculum. Acad Med. 1998;73:403–407.

Becoming a Consummate Clinician: What Every Student, House Officer, and Hospital Practitioner Needs to Know, First Edition.
Ary L. Goldberger and Zachary D. Goldberger.
© 2012 Wiley-Blackwell. Published 2012 by John Wiley & Sons, Inc.

Krupat E, Pelletier S, Alexander EK, Hirsh D, Ogur B, Schwartzstein R. Can changes in the principal clinical year prevent the erosion of students' patient-centered beliefs? Acad Med. 2009;84:582–586.

Moore GE. Cramming more components into integrated circuits. Electronics. 1965;38: 114–117.

National Commission on Terrorist Attacks upon the United States. The 9/11 Commission Report. New York: W.W. Norton, 2004.

Nobel Lectures, Physiology or Medicine, 1942–62. Amsterdam: Elsevier, 1962.

Chapter 1   How (Not) to Present a Patient History

Corda RS, Burke HB, Horowitz HW. Adherence to prescription medications among medical professionals. South Med J. 2000;93:585–589.

http://www.ihi.org/IHI/Topics/PatientSafety/MedicationSystems/Literature/.

Neeman N, Isaac T, Leveille S, Dimonda C, Shin JY, Aronson MD, Freedman SD. Improving doctor–patient communication in the outpatient setting using a facilitation tool: a preliminary study. Int J Qual Health Care. 2011;Dec (Epub ahead of print).

Osterberg L, Blaschke T. Adherence to medication. N Engl J Med. 2005;353:487–497.

Chapter 2   Reexamining the Physical Exam

Constant J. Bedside Cardiology, 5th ed. Philadelphia: Lippincott Williams & Wilkins, 1999.

Cook DJ, Simel DL. The rational clinical examination: Does this patient have abnormal central venous pressure? JAMA. 1996;275:630–634.

Gawande A. Naked. N Engl J Med. 2005;353:645–648.

Jauhar S. The demise of the physical exam. N Engl J Med. 2006;354:548–551.

Ma I, Tierney LM. Name that murmur—eponyms for the astute auscultician. N Engl J Med. 2010;363:2164–2168.

Max J. The lost art of the physical exam. Yale Med. 2009;Winter:31–35.

McGee S. Evidence-Based Physical Diagnosis, 2nd ed. St. Louis, MO: W.B. Saunders, 2007.

Simel DL, Rennie D, eds. The Rational Clinical Examination: Evidence-Based Clinical Diagnosis. New York, McGraw-Hill, 2009.

Treadway K. Heart sounds. N Engl J Med. 2006;354:1112–1113.

Chapter 3   How (Not) to Order and Present Lab Tests

Fischbach FT, Dunning MB III. Manual of Laboratory and Diagnostic Tests, 8th ed. Philadelphia: Lippincott Williams & Wilkins, 2008.

Mann EA, Mora AG, Pidcoke HF, et al. Glycemic control in the burn intensive care unit: focus on the role of anemia in glucose measurement. J Diabetes Sci Technol. 2009;3:1319–1329.

Chapter 4 Seeing Is (Almost) Believing: The Importance of Reviewing Data

Gierada DS, Pilgram TK, Ford M, et al. Lung cancer: interobserver agreement on interpretation of pulmonary findings at low-dose CT screening. Radiology. 2008;246:265–272.

Gow RM, Barrowman NJ, Lai L, Moher D. A review of five cardiology journals found that observer variability of measured variables was infrequently reported. J Clin Epidemiol. 2008;61:394–401.

McGinn T, Wyer PC, Newman TB, Keitz S, Leipzig R, For GG. Evidence-Based Medicine Teaching Tips Working Group. Tips for learners of evidence-based medicine: 3. Measures of observer variability (kappa statistic). CMAJ. 2004;17:1369–1373. Erratum in: CMAJ. 2005;18:173.

Spodick DH, Bishop RL. Computer treason: intraobserver variability of an electrocardiographic computer system. Am J Cardiol. 1997;80:102–103.

Chapter 5 "Worsts First": How to Frame a Differential Diagnosis

Croskerry P. The importance of cognitive errors in diagnosis and strategies to minimize them. Acad Med. 2003;78:775–780.

Fauci AS, Braunwald EB, Kasper DL, et al. Harrison's Principles of Internal Medicine, 17th ed. New York: McGraw-Hill, 2008.

Silen W. Cope's Early Diagnosis of the Acute Abdomen, 22nd ed. Oxford, UK: Oxford University Press, 2010.

Chapter 6 Clinical Queries: Asking the 3½ Key Questions

Gladwell M. Blink: The Power of Thinking Without Thinking. New York: Little, Brown, 2005.

Goldberger AL. Clinical Electrocardiography: A Simplified Approach, 7th ed. St. Louis, MO: Mosby/Elsevier, 2006.

Groopman J. How Doctors Think. Boston: Houghton Mifflin, 2007.

Marshall BJ, Warren JR. Unidentified curved bacillus on gastric epithelium in active chronic gastritis. Lancet. 1983;1:1273–1275.

Chapter 7 $E = mc^3$: Error Reduction Equals Motivation Times Communication to the Power of 3

Aronson MD, Neeman N, Carbo A, Tess AV, Yang JJ, Folcarelli P, Sands KF, Zeidel ML. A model for quality improvement programs in academic departments of medicine. Am J Med. 2008;121:922–929.

Bell SK, Moorman DW, Delbanco T. Improving the patient, family, and clinician experience after harmful events: the "when things go wrong" curriculum. Acad Med. 2010;85:1010–1017.

Bordage G. Why did I miss the diagnosis? Some cognitive explanation and educational implications. Acad Med. 1999;74:S138–S143.

Delbanco T, Bell SK. Guilty, afraid, and alone—struggling with medical error. N Engl J Med. 2007;357:1682–1683.

Fleischut PM, Evans AS, Nugent WC. Ten years after the IOM report: engaging residents in quality and patient safety by creating a house staff quality council. Am J Qual. 2011;26:89–94.

Graber ML, Franklin N, Gordon R. Diagnostic error in internal medicine. Arch Intern Med. 2005;165:1493–1499.

Huang GC, Newman LR, Tess AV, Schwartzstein RM. Teaching patient safety: conference proceedings and consensus statements of the Millennium Conference 2009. Teach Learn Med. 2011;23:172–178.

Irby DM, Cooke M, O'Brien BC. Calls for reform of medical education by the Carnegie Foundation for the Advancement of Teaching: 1910 and 2010. Acad Med. 2010;85:220–227.

Kohn KT, Corrigan JM, Donaldson MS. To Err Is Human: Building a Safer Health System. Washington, DC: National Academy Press, 1999.

Leape L, Lawthers AG, Brennan TA, Johnson WG. Preventing medical injury. Qual Rev Bull. 1993;19:144–149.

Roberts DH, Gilmartin GS, Neeman N, Schulze JE, Cannistraro S, Ngo LH, Aronson MD, Weiss JW. Design and measurement of quality improvement indicators in ambulatory pulmonary care: creating a "culture of quality" in an academic pulmonary division. Chest. 2009;136:1134–1140.

Zeidel M. Systematic quality improvement in medicine: Everyone can do it. RMMJ. 2011;2:1–7. http://www.rmmj.org.il/userimages/70/0/PublishFiles/70Article.pdf.

Chapter 8 Evidence-Based Medicine: What and Where Is the Evidence?

Note: An enormous amount has been written about evidence-based medicine (EBM). The discussion here is intended to call attention to some less emphasized aspects and also foster a critical and neutral reexamination of the evidence-based process so that in the best spirit of EBM, nothing gets taken for granted, including the process and products of EBM themselves.

Dubey RK, Imthurn B, Zacharia LC, Jackson EK. Hormone replacement therapy and cardiovascular disease: What went wrong and where do we go from here? Hypertension. 2004;44:789–795.

Epstein AE, DiMarco JP, Ellenbogen KA, et al. ACC/AHA/HRS 2008 Guidelines for Device-Based Therapy of Cardiac Rhythm Abnormalities: A report of the American College of Cardiology/American Heart Association Task Force. J Am Coll Cardiol. 2008;51:61–62.

Evidence-Based Medicine Working Group. Evidence-based medicine: A new approach to teaching the practice of medicine. JAMA. 1992;268:2420–2425.

Goldberger AL, Amaral LAN, Glass L, Hausdorff JM, Ivanov PCh, Mark RG, Mietus JE, Moody GB, Peng CK, Stanley HE. PhysioBank, PhysioToolkit, and PhysioNet: components of a new research resource for complex physiologic signals. Circulation. 2000;101:e215–e220. http://circ.ahajournals.org/cgi/content/full/101/23/e215.

Goldberger ZD, Goldberger AL. Therapeutic ranges of serum digoxin concentrations in patients with heart failure. Am J Cardiol. 2012;109:1818–1821.

Guyatt G, Gutterman D, Baumann MH, et al. Grading strength of recommendations and quality of evidence in clinical guidelines: report from an American College of Chest Physicians task force. Chest. 2006;129:174–181.

Ioannides JAP. Why most published research findings are false. PLoS Med. 2005;2:e124.

Kent DM, Hayward RA. Limitations of applying summary results of clinical trials to individual patients: the need for risk stratification. JAMA. 2007;298:1209–1212.

Malterud K. The art and science of clinical knowledge: evidence beyond measures and numbers. Lancet. 2001;358:397–400.

Straus SE, McAlister FA. Evidence-based medicine: a commentary on common criticisms. CMAJ. 2000;163:837–841.

Chapter 9   Caution! Dangerous Biomedical Semantics at Work

Goldberger AL. Non-linear dynamics for physicians: chaos theory, fractals, and complexity at the bedside. Lancet. 1996;347:1312–1314.

Strebhardt K, Ullrich A. Paul Ehrlich's magic bullet concept: 100 years of progress. Nat Rev Cancer. 2008;8:473–480.

The Cardiac Arrhythmia Suppression Trial (CAST) Investigators. Preliminary report: effect of encainide and flecainide on mortality in a randomized trial of arrhythmia suppression after myocardial infarction. N Engl J Med. 1989;321:406–412.

Chapter 10   Some Second Opinions: Outliers, Hoofbeats, and Sutton's (Flawed) Law

Hunter K. "Don't think zebras": uncertainty, interpretation, and the place of paradox in clinical education. Theor Med. 1996;17:225–241.

Kassirer JP, Kopelman RI. A fatal flaw in Sutton's law. Hosp Pract. 1986;65–74.

Rytand D. Sutton's or Dock's law? N Engl J Med. 1980;302:972.

Sutton W, Lynn E. Where the Money Was: The Memoirs of a Bank Robber. New York: Viking, 1976.

Chapter 11 A Sixfold Path: From Data to Knowledge to Understanding

André D, Fernand G. Sherlock Holmes: an expert's view of expertise. Br J Psychol. 2008;99(Pt 1):109–125.

Daley BJ, Torre DM. Concept maps in medical education: an analytical literature review. Med Educ. 2010;44:440–448.

Friedlander MJ, Andrews L, Armstrong EG, Aschenbrenner C, Kass JS, Ogden P, Schwartzstein R, Viggiano TR. What can medical education learn from the neurobiology of learning? Acad Med. 2011;86:415–420.

Guerrero APS. Mechanistic case diagramming: a tool for problem-based learning. Acad Med. 2001;76:385–389.

Mennin S. Self-organisation, integration and curriculum in the complex world of medical education. Med Educ. 2010;44:20–30.

Naghshineh S, Hafler JP, Miller AR. Formal art observation training improves medical students' visual diagnostic skills. J Gen Intern Med. 2008;23:9971–9977.

Chapter 12 What Is Disease? What Is Health?

Aird WC, ed. Endothelial Biomedicine. Cambridge, UK: Cambridge University Press, 2007.

Barabási AL, Gulbahce N, Loscalzo J. Network medicine: a network-based approach to human disease. Nat Rev Genet. 2011;12:56–68.

Folkman J, Kalluri R. Cancer without disease. Nature. 2004;427:787.

Fried LP, Tangen CM, Walson J, et al. Frailty in older adults: evidence for a phenotype. J Gerontol A Biol Sci Med Sci. 2001;56:M146–M157.

Go AS, Hylek EM, Phillips KA, et al. Prevalence of diagnosed atrial fibrillation in adults. JAMA. 2001;285:2370–2375.

Hales CN, Barker DJ. Type 2 (non-insulin-dependent) diabetes mellitus: the thrifty phenotype hypothesis. Diabetologia. 1992;35:595–601.

Leor J, Kloner RA. The Northridge earthquake as a trigger for acute myocardial infarction. Am J Cardiol. 1996;77:1230–1232.

Lipsitz LA. The dynamics of stability: the physiologic basis of functional health and frailty. J Gerontol Biol Sci. 2002;57A:B115–B125.

Lynch JW, Kaplan GA, Shema SJ. Cumulative impact of sustained economic hardship on physical, cognitive, psychological, and social functioning. N Engl J Med. 1997;337:1889–1895.

Petersdorf RG, Beeson PB. Fever of unexplained origin: report on 100 cases. Medicine (Baltimore). 1961;40:1–30.

Rosenberg CE. Contested boundaries: psychiatry, disease, and diagnosis. Perspect Biol Med. 2006;49:407–424.

Steinberg JS, Arshad A, Kowalski M, et al. Increased incidence of life-threatening ventricular arrhythmias in implantable defibrillator patients after the World Trade Center attack. J Am Coll Cardiol. 2004;44:1261–1264.

Tomes N. Epidemic entertainments: disease and popular culture in early-twentieth-century America. Am Lit Hist. 2002;14:625–652.

SOME OTHER USEFUL RESOURCES FOR CLINICAL AND SCIENTIFIC REASONING SKILLS

Academic Medicine (excellent general resource, including Point–Counterpoint articles)

American Journal of Medicine (including articles on the physical exam and on clinical effectiveness)

Annals of Medicine (especially Academia and the Profession; In the Balance)

Journal of General Internal Medicine (especially Innovations in Education; Innovations in Clinical Research)

New England Journal of Medicine (especially Interactive Medical Cases; Clinical Problem-Solving)

Scientific American (many discoveries in medicine come from far afield)

INDEX

Page references followed by e denote exhibits; those followed by f denote figures; those followed by t denote tables.

Becoming a Consummate Clinician: What Every Student, House Officer, and Hospital Practitioner Needs to Know, First Edition.
Ary L. Goldberger and Zachary D. Goldberger.
© 2012 Wiley-Blackwell. Published 2012 by John Wiley & Sons, Inc.